Gayle's Feel-Good Foods

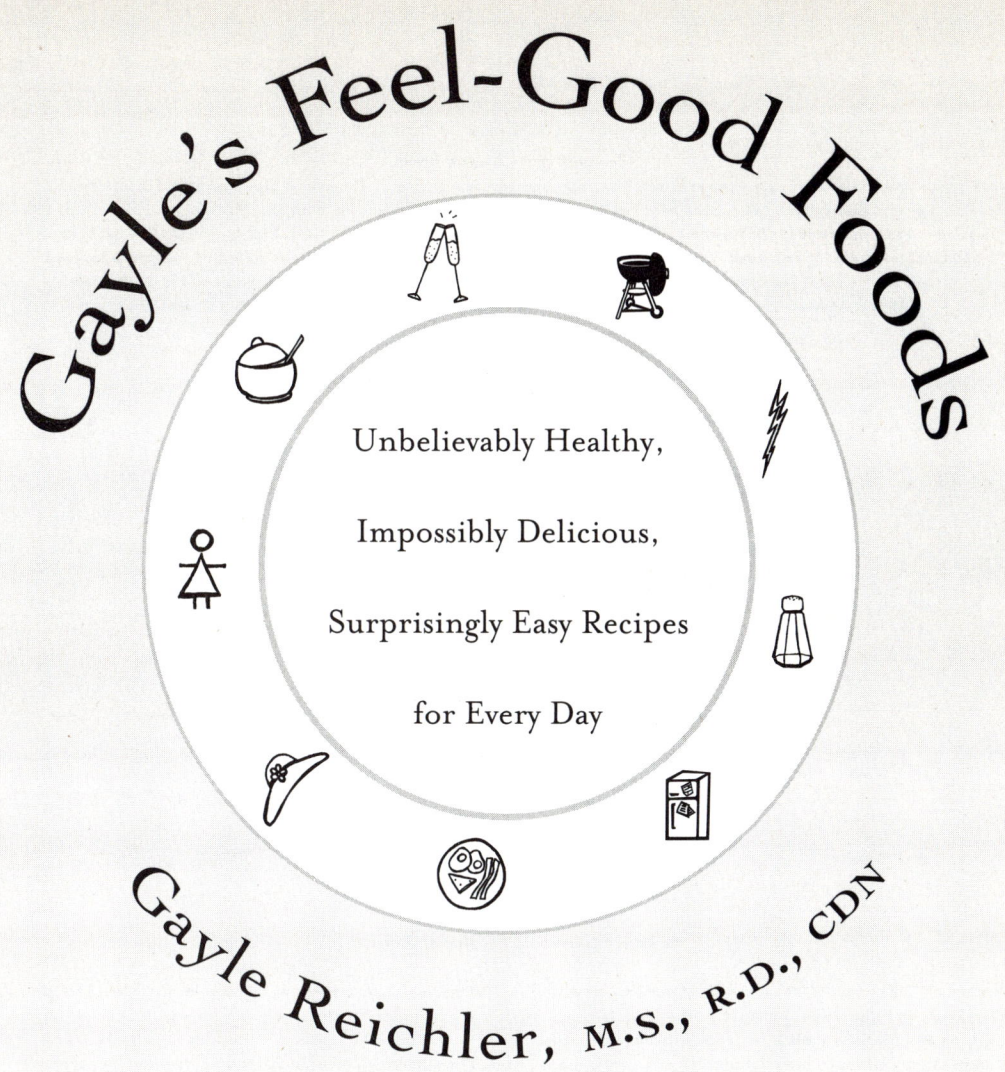

Gayle's Feel-Good Foods

Unbelievably Healthy, Impossibly Delicious, Surprisingly Easy Recipes for Every Day

Gayle Reichler, M.S., R.D., CDN

Avery

a member of Penguin Group (USA) Inc.

New York

Published by the Penguin Group
Penguin Group (USA) Inc., 375 Hudson Street, New York, New York 10014, USA · Penguin Group (Canada), 10 Alcorn Avenue, Toronto, Ontario, Canada M4V 3B2 (a division of Pearson Penguin Canada Inc.) · Penguin Books Ltd, 80 Strand, London WC2R 0RL, England · Penguin Ireland, 25 St Stephen's Green, Dublin 2, Ireland (a division of Penguin Books Ltd) · Penguin Group (Australia), 250 Camberwell Road, Camberwell, Victoria 3124, Australia (a division of Pearson Australia Group Pty Ltd) · Penguin Books India, 11 Community Centre, Panchsheel Park, New Delhi—110 017, India · Penguin Group (NZ), Cnr Airborne and Rosedale Roads, Albany, Auckland 1310, New Zealand (a division of Pearson New Zealand Ltd) · Penguin Books (South Africa) (Pty) Ltd, 24 Sturdee Avenue, Rosebank, Johannesburg 2196, South Africa

Penguin Books Ltd, Registered Offices: 80 Strand, London WC2R 0RL, England

Copyright © 2004 by Gayle Reichler
All rights reserved. No part of this book may be reproduced, scanned, or distributed in any printed or electronic form without permission. Please do not participate in or encourage piracy of copyrighted materials in violation of the author's rights. Purchase only authorized editions.
Published simultaneously in Canada

Library of Congress Cataloging-in-Publication Data

Reichler, Gayle.
Gayle's feel-good foods: unbelievably healthy, impossibly delicious, surprisingly easy recipes for every day / Gayle Reichler.
    p.   cm.
Includes index.
ISBN 1-58333-199-9
1. Low-fat diet—Recipes.   I. Title.
RM237.7.R45   2004
641.5'6384—dc22   2004054414

Printed in the United States of America
1 3 5 7 9 10 8 6 4 2

Book design and illustrations by Meighan Cavanaugh

Neither the publisher nor the author is engaged in rendering professional advice or services to the individual reader. The ideas, procedures, and suggestions contained in this book are not intended as a substitute for consulting with your physician. All matters regarding health require medical supervision. Neither the author nor the publisher shall be liable or responsible for any loss, injury, or damage allegedly arising from any information or suggestion in this book. The opinions expressed in this book represent the personal views of the author and not of the publisher.

While the author has made every effort to provide accurate telephone numbers and Internet addresses at the time of publication, neither the publisher nor the author assumes any responsibility for errors or for changes that occur after publication.

Most Avery books are available at special quantity discounts for bulk purchase for sales promotions, premiums, fund-raising, and educational needs. Special books or book excerpts also can be created to fit specific needs. For details, write Penguin Group (USA) Inc. Special Markets, 375 Hudson Street, New York, NY 10014.

*To my husband, Doug, and

our son, Harrison*

Acknowledgments

My love of food and recipe development has always been nurtured by my clients' desire for tasty, healthy foods that are easy to prepare. This has spurred me on to create low-fat favorites from traditional recipes. A big thank-you to all my clients whose desire for great-tasting, healthy food has given me the challenge to rise beyond their expectations with tasty, healthy solutions that have led to many of the recipes in this book.

In addition, the recipes in *Gayle's Feel-Good Foods* would not have been written if it weren't for the feedback from my friends, family, and clients who have tasted, tested, and critiqued my recipes. A special thanks goes in particular to Ann Boroweic, Kathy Buergert, Kathleen Flaherty, Rosalyn Stone, and Christine Wagner. Plus to those who tried the recipes—the brave taste testers—my husband, family, and friends: a special thanks for being available with an open mind and a big appetite.

I would also like to acknowledge the support I was always given by the institutions where I taught cooking—the New School Cooking School and New York University, where I taught food science. Additionally, I would like to thank the spas where I regularly give lectures and teach cooking—Canyon Ranch, Exhale, and Avon. Plus, special recognition goes to the French Culinary Institute, where I received my foundation as a chef in their Culinary Arts program.

Last but not least, this book would not have made it to press if it weren't for the terrific team at Penguin—Kristen Jennings, Megan Newman, and Kate Stark. Plus, my dedicated team—Lisa Altman and Cindy Bressler of Smash Arts and Laurie Pollock—as well as my book agents at Dorie Simmonds, Lmtd.

Contents

Introduction *1*

1. Using the Recipes to Lose Weight and Feel Good

   5

2. Breakfast

   27

3. Appetizers and Party Foods

   51

4. Soups and Chili

   73

5. Salads

93

6. Sandwiches

119

7. Entrées

129

8. Sides

199

9. Desserts

227

Appendix I
Quick Guides for Cooking Beans and Grains   *257*

Appendix II
Chart of Measurements   *263*

Resources for Ingredients   *267*

Index   *269*

Gayle's Feel-Good Foods

■ ■ ■

Introduction

I am excited to share my recipes for *Feel-Good Foods* with you. As a nutritionist and chef, my focus has been to create recipes that both please the palate and satisfy the requirements for low-fat, healthy fare. I have always welcomed this challenge, because we are what we eat, so in order to be healthy you need to eat healthfully. But, you also want to enjoy your food, or why eat it? So I put my skills together to create these mouthwatering favorites that you can feel safe eating if you are health conscious, want to lose weight, or just feel good feeding your family. With my recipes you will be able to satisfy your appetite, taste buds, and waistline. I am hoping that just by knowing that all the foods you will be cooking are good for you, that you will not only feel good, but enjoy indulging with every bite!

It has always been a frustration for me that the general belief is that nutritious eating needs to taste "healthy" or "granola," like you are eating tree bark, because I know this is not true. In fact, a common obstacle I have had to face is that people don't believe healthy, low-fat foods can taste as decadent as their high-fat counterparts. Given this challenge, I have devoted my cooking career to dispelling this myth with my surprisingly delicious low-fat chocolates and recipes. Sometimes, I have even had to fool my dinner guests by giving them a meal and then telling them how healthy it was and how many calories and fat grams they saved. Everyone is always pleasantly surprised.

Luckily, I also have my Gayle's Miracle Perfect Chocolate Truffles to stand behind as a true testament to the quality and indulgence low-fat foods can have. This year my truffle, Gayle's Miracles: The Perfect Chocolate Truffle, won Upscale Gourmet Candy Product of the Year, awarded by *Professional Candy Buyer* magazine. And, it was the only candy out of the top five nominees that was healthy, with only 30 calories, 1 gram of fat, and low in sugar. Now, people who normally don't trust low-fat meals are trusting me to produce foods they will like. Using my recipes, you too can fool your family and friends and feel assured at the same time that you are providing yourself and others with nutritious foods that won't pack on the pounds.

Contrary to what you may think, preparing healthy food that is also tasty isn't difficult. It simply involves learning a few easy techniques, which you can use every time you cook. First, accentuating the full flavors of fresh foods by choosing and combining the right ingredients and using ingenious low-fat cooking techniques will bring out the full taste and texture of foods. Next, learning basic nutrition principles to help you combine the energy nutrients of proteins, fats, and carbohydrates will allow you to create nutritionally balanced meals that can even help you lose weight. Soon, you will be able to put together my tips for cooking and nutrition and apply your skill and knowledge to converting your family favorites to new healthy alternatives.

My hope is that this book can become your "bible" for healthy cooking and that you enjoy the foods you cook from this book so much you won't need to cook any other way. I have placed special features throughout the book to help you meet your health goals, including:

- "Gayle's Feel-Good Facts," which contain helpful nutritional tips and facts
- Nutritional analysis of each recipe
- Guidelines on how to curb cravings so that you can achieve your goal weight
- Calorie-controlled weight-loss menus using the recipes in this book

- Icons accompanying each recipe that will allow you to quickly determine which recipes fit with your lifestyle needs. These simple icons reveal what foods to cook if you only have twenty minutes, meals that can be frozen, and recipes for when you are entertaining friends and more
- "Quick Tips" throughout to make the recipes as easy as possible for you to cook

The recipes draw on flavors from a variety of cultures. The ingredients listed are those you can easily find in your supermarket or local stores. But since eating healthy is also about the quality of the ingredients you use, there are charts that cover questions about what fish is safe to eat, what oils are best to use, and how and when to use sugar or a sugar alternative in your cooking. In the appendix I have included a list of distributors of ingredients that you can purchase by mail order or online.

You will have all the tools and recipes you need to ensure you are doing your best to cook healthy meals that will wow anyone. The best part is no one will believe the food is also healthy. But they will thank you for it when they do.

Eat and be well with every bite!
Gayle

Using the Recipes to Lose Weight and Feel Good

There is no question, delicious food will make you feel good. Just to eat it is a great experience. Now with Gayle's Feel-Good recipes, you can both take pleasure in your eating experience and indulge in the fact that you are doing something good for yourself by eating low-fat, healthy meals. The recipes taste so good, you will not realize they are also good for you. Whether it is a low-fat version of a traditional favorite or a new recipe you want to try, all the recipes have been created so that they are packed with flavor and healthy ingredients.

As a registered dietitian, I can assure you that you can also feel good because you will be taking care of yourself and your health when you indulge in *Gayle's Feel-Good Foods*. You can feel good eating the foods in this book because the recipes are not only low in fat, but they are also reduced in refined flours and sugar, as well as sodium. Attention to the nutrition content of the recipes is especially important because dietary fat has been linked to many diseases including cancer, diabetes, and heart disease and processed flours and sugars may be associated with diabetes and obesity. Since many people who have high blood pressure are also watching their salt intake, I reduced the salt to only what was necessary to use in each recipe. If you are not salt sensitive or watching your sodium intake, feel free to add more salt to your foods.

Gayle's Feel-Good Foods will help you manage your weight and health because the recipes are designed to give you a satisfying eating experience, eliminating the boredom and insatiable cravings that often come from eating meals that are unappealing or what my clients refer to as "diet food." In many healthy recipes you can tell by the taste which have reduced fat, but I use a flavor-layering technique that promotes both variety in taste and textures, so your mouth doesn't miss the qualities fat usually adds by carrying the flavors and scent and adding mouth-feel.

Losing Weight with *Gayle's Feel-Good Foods*

When you eat more than your body needs you will gain weight. Contrary to the teachings put forth in many popular diets, there is not one nutrient that is particularly to blame for weight loss or weight gain. Gaining weight can happen from any nutrient—eating too much carbohydrate, protein, or fat can do it. However, since pound for pound fat has more than two times the calories (energy) than proteins or carbohydrates, eating too much fat in your diet will easily give you more calories than your body can use and you will often gain weight. But no need to worry, my Feel-Good recipes are designed to fill you up on less calories, because the meals are low in fat and high in fiber. High fiber foods help add to your feeling of satiation, because they provide a feeling of fullness, while at the same time fiber is also good for your health. A diet that is high in fiber means that it is made with whole grains, fruits, and vegetables, which can help prevent some cancers, reduce your cholesterol, and maintain good digestion.

Below are sample weight-loss menus that tell you how many servings of different types of meals you can have each day. These menu plans emphasize how to combine foods throughout the day so you can feel good eating to meet your body's needs and achieving your ideal weight. By using the menu layouts, you will see how easy it can be to both eat and lose weight at the same time.

You will notice that vegetable portions are unlimited because they are so low in calories. So enjoy vegetable soup, or cooked, roasted, or steamed vegetables anytime. These tasty menu plans will make you feel like you are "dining" instead of "dieting," and eating will be enjoyable as you meet your weight goals.

Along with the foods, be sure to drink plenty of water—32 ounces—throughout the day to stay well hydrated. Dehydration can mask hunger and it will also make you feel sluggish. Beware of drinking caffeinated beverages that can dehydrate you and counter your weight loss by causing you to crave sweets. Be sure when drinking caffeinated or alcoholic beverages to add at least two additional glasses of water in your day to rehydrate.

If you are interested in losing weight you can also employ an eating strategy that helps you feel more satisfied with less food and reduces cravings. The strategy involves mixing the nutrient groups of proteins, carbohydrates, and fats in each meal. By mixing the nutrient groups of proteins, carbohydrates, and fats in each meal, your body stays full longer. This happens because carbohydrates are digested first, then proteins, then fats. So, by combining the nutrient groups you eat at every meal your body has more to work with and you can be more satisfied with less food. A basic "recipe" to use is to always mix the carbohydrate group with either protein, fat, or both. The sidebar can help you distinguish between the food groups. Also, the more processed the carbohydrate the quicker it is digested and raises your blood sugar, both factors that can contribute to feelings of hunger. To learn which foods are in each nutrient group and which carbohydrates are more likely to raise your blood sugar faster, see below.

The Effect of Different Food Groups on Blood Sugar

The following list of foods is arranged by the degree to which they affect your blood sugar. Carbohydrates rank at the top of the list, ranging from highly refined sugars that raise your blood sugar the most to beans and vegetables, which only raise your

(continued)

blood sugar moderately. Plant fats and lean proteins do not raise your blood sugar in the same way as carbohydrates.

CARBOHYDRATES
Sugar and other sweeteners, soda, candy, cakes, cookies, and pies
Fruit juice, dried fruit
White bread, white-flour pasta, potatoes, refined breakfast cereals, processed flour products
Whole fruit
Whole-grain products such as breads, pastas, cereals, crackers, popcorn
Beans, lentils, low-fat dairy (these products contain protein, but are mainly comprised of carbohydrates)
Vegetables

PLANT FATS
Nuts, seeds, oils, nut butters, avocado, olives

LEAN PROTEIN
Fish, poultry without skin, lean beef, pork, game, beans, egg whites, and soy products

Women's Sample Menu Layout for Weight Loss
(Approximately 1200 calories)

Breakfast: 1 serving of a breakfast recipe, that is, 240 calories or less
1 fruit (if there is no fruit in your breakfast recipe)
Water, herbal tea, decaf tea, or coffee
Lunch: 1 serving of a lunch recipe (sandwich, salad, bean soup, or an entrée, 300 calories or less)
2 or more side vegetables (salad, vegetable soup, or cooked vegetables)

Snack:	1 piece of fruit or 1 appetizer, up to 100 calories
Dinner:	1 entrée serving, 400 calories or less
	2 or more vegetables, grilled, roasted, or steamed
	A glass of wine or 1 drink if desired
Dessert:	1 serving of a dessert or 1 piece of fruit, 200 calories or less

*Drink water, herbal teas, or mineral water throughout the day

Men's Sample Menu Layout for Weight Loss
(Approximately 2000 calories)

Breakfast:	1 serving of a breakfast recipe, 240 calories or less
	1 fruit
	Water, herbal tea, decaf tea, or coffee
Lunch:	1 serving of a lunch recipe (can be a sandwich, salad, and bean soup, or an entrée, 400 calories or less)
	2 or more side vegetables (salad, vegetable soup, or cooked vegetables)
	1 serving of grain/starch side dish
Snack:	1 snack recipe or a piece of fruit or 1 appetizer serving
Dinner:	1 to 2 entrée servings, 500 calories or less
	2 or more vegetables
	1 serving of a grain or starch side dish
	A glass of wine or one drink if desired
Dessert:	1 serving of a dessert (if you didn't have it as a snack), 300 calories or less, or a piece of fruit

*Drink water, herbal teas, or mineral water throughout the day

Sample Weight Loss Menu Using Gayle's Feel-Good Recipes

Breakfast: 1 to 2 servings of Almond Oatmeal Pancakes with a cup of fruit salad with yogurt sauce

Lunch: A cup of Vegetable Soup,
Roasted Salmon Salad with buttermilk dressing

Snack: 1 serving Hummus and Roasted Vegetables or Vegetable Soup (Vegetable Soup is unlimited) or Herbed Cheese Spread (1 serving) on whole grain crackers with fruit on the side

Dinner: Garden Salad with Roasted Vegetables and Balsamic Dressing
Yummy Low-Fat Spinach Lasagna (1–2 servings)
A glass of wine or 1 drink if desired

Dessert: A slice of I Can't Believe It's Low-Fat Cheesecake

*Drink water, herbal teas, or mineral water throughout the day

Nutrition Guidelines Used to Develop the Recipes

The recipes have been created using fresh, whole ingredients that you can easily find at your local supermarket—unsaturated fats (oil, nuts, seeds, olives, avocado), lean proteins (fish, seafood, poultry, game, and meats), and carbohydrates (whole fruits, vegetables, beans, and grains). Below is a list of the ingredients used and their nutritional benefits.

FATS

A diet low in total fat and in particular saturated fat and hydrogenated fat (margarine) will be less likely to raise your cholesterol, clog your arteries, and cause health risks. Therefore, all the recipes in this book are based on 3 grams or less of fat, and meals or combination foods have 30 percent of total fat or less per serving.

Fats can be categorized as either "good" or "bad." Bad fats are saturated fats and hydrogenated fats. Saturated fats typically come from animal and dairy sources. According to the American Heart Association, your diet should only consist of 10 percent saturated fat or less. I designed *Gayle's Feel-Good Foods* using mainly unsaturated "good" fats—those originally derived from plants and composed of unsaturated fats that stay liquid in your body and promote health. Omega-3 and omega-6 are unsaturated fats that are essential to the diet because the body cannot make them. In the American diet we consume plenty of omega-6 fats from vegetable oil, but not enough omega-3 fats. So, I designed these recipes to encourage the consumption of omega-3 fats. Some recipes are so chock-full of healthy fats that they will have more than 3 grams of fat per serving. But, that's OK, because it is all good fat that is beneficial to eat.

However, there are some instances in a recipe where it made the most sense to use a very limited amount of butter so as not to sacrifice on texture and mouth-feel of a recipe. This small amount of saturated fat in a recipe is the exception rather than the rule and has been applied to dessert recipes only, and it is well within the acceptable limits set by the American Heart Association.

BAD FATS	GOOD FATS	
Saturated fats	**Polyunsaturated fats**	**Monounsaturated fats**
Butter	Safflower oil	Olive oil
Fat marbling on animal meats (beef, pork, lamb, veal)	Sunflower oil	Canola oil
Dairy fat—whole milk, cheeses, cream, ice cream	Corn oil	Peanut oil
		(continued)

BAD FATS	GOOD FATS	
Saturated fats	Polyunsaturated fats	Monounsaturated fats
Skin on poultry	Seeds: flax, sesame, sunflower, pumpkin	Avocado
Tropical oils—coconut and palm kernel oil	Nuts: walnuts, cashews, pecans, pine nuts	Olives
Lard	Fish—oily cold water varieties—salmon, trout, sardines, halibut	Nuts: almonds, peanuts

Sugars

All of my Feel-Good recipes were created with a limited amount of sugars and where possible, refined sugars such as table sugars and brown sugar were replaced with fructose, maple syrup, fruit-juice concentrate, or honey, which are less likely to raise your blood sugars and make you hungry. While you do not need to deprive yourself completely of sweets, it is important for health reasons to focus on low-fat desserts to limit your intake of saturated "bad" fats. Granulated sugar and brown sugar are used sparingly in order to capture flavor and texture when necessary, to preserve the quality of the recipe. If you are a diabetic, look for desserts that are sweetened only by fruit, honey, or fructose, as they will be easier to have when you are managing your blood sugar levels.

Grains and Starch

Whole grains are grains that have not been milled and stripped of their bran and germ in processing. They are the healthiest grains to use, because they still contain additional vitamins and are higher in fiber than their processed counterparts. Processed grains are often white and found in items such as pasta, bagels, white bread, white rice, and processed cereals and crackers. If you eat a meal mainly of processed grain products, it will go through your digestive system quickly and before you know it you will be hungry for more food. Processed grains are also more likely to raise your blood sugar levels, promoting hunger.

This doesn't mean you need to cut out processed grains entirely. After all, when you go to a restaurant it is not always easy to find whole grains. Just be smart about how you eat them and keep them limited in your overall eating plan. Starches include beans and legumes and starchy vegetables, which include potatoes, corn, peas, winter orange squash, beans, and plantains. Enjoy starches as part of a healthy diet. They are low in calories and add great variety to any diet.

Gayle's Feel-Good Facts

Myth: Grains, starches, and fats like peanut butter are fattening.
Contrary to popular belief, these foods are not fattening. It is overeating them that makes you fat. So enjoy a balance of foods every day and stay satisfied longer!

VEGETABLES AND FRUITS

Vegetables that are not considered "starchy" are to be eaten in abundance because they provide you with numerous protective nutrients and they are low in calories and high in fiber. Vegetable recipes included in Feel-Good Foods are in dips, soups, and side dishes. To get the most nutrients from your fruits and vegetables, aim for a variety of color when eating and cooking—the red, orange, dark green, and blue foods are packed with protective antioxidant benefits. Organic produce is often more flavorful because it is ripened longer in the fields. Below is a chart of power fruits and vegetables and their antioxidants.

FOODS RICH IN ANTIOXIDANTS AND OTHER VITAMINS

Carotenoids	Vitamin C	Vitamin E	Folate
Vegetables			
Asparagus	Broccoli	Artichoke	Asparagus
Broccoli	Brussels Sprouts	Asparagus	Broccoli
Carrots	Cabbage	Broccoli	Beets
Dark green, leafy vegetables (Arugula, Chicory, Dandelion Greens, Kale, Mustard Greens, Spinach)	Cauliflower	Dark green, leafy vegetables (Collard Greens, Kale, Spinach, Swiss Chard)	Cauliflower
	Chili Peppers		Dark green, leafy vegetables (Collard Greens, Kale, Spinach)
	Dark green, leafy vegetables (Collard Greens, Kale, Mustard and Turnip Greens)	Onions	
Pumpkin			Seaweed
Tomatoes	Peppers (green and red)		
	Radishes		
Fruits			
Apricot	Grapefruit	Avocado	Avocado
Cantaloupe	Kiwi	Blueberries	Banana
Mango	Orange	Mango	Blackberries
Nectarine	Papaya	Olives	Mango
Papaya	Strawberries	Papaya	Papaya

Gayle's Feel-Good Facts

The fruits and vegetables with the most pesticides at this point in time are strawberries, grapes, cherries, apples, pears, peaches, spinach, sweet bell peppers, and lettuce. According to the USDA, 23 percent of organic produce has pesticide residue, whereas 73 percent of conventional produce contains pesticides. The organic produce contains some pesticides because it is often farmed next to or near conventional produce and the air and wind carries the pesticides onto the plants. When possible, try to choose produce that is organic to limit your exposure to pesticide chemicals.

PROTEINS—LEAN MEATS, FISH, SHELLFISH, POULTRY, EGGS, SOY AND BEANS

Animal protein is high in saturated fat, which raises your cholesterol. To avoid this unhealthy element, the recipes in this book use leaner proteins. When choosing lean proteins, you want to look for the loin or round cuts of meats, skinless poultry, and any fish or shellfish. If you have high cholesterol, you will want to avoid the yolks of eggs and focus on egg whites. Soy products and beans are fine sources of protein that provide healthy fats and do not need to be eaten in their low-fat varieties.

TYPE OF MEAT	CUTS TO LOOK FOR
Beef	Eye round, top round, tip round, top sirloin, top loin, tenderloin, flank (trimmed of visible fat)
Pork	Tenderloin, boneless sirloin chop, top loin roast, boneless top loin chop, rib chop, boneless rib roast, sirloin roast, ham
Ground meat and poultry	95% lean beef, ground pork loin, ground turkey, ground chicken *(continued)*

TYPE OF MEAT	CUTS TO LOOK FOR
Poultry	Skinless chicken breast, skinless dark meat, roasted hen, chicken, or turkey eaten without the skin.
Veal	Loin, medallions
Lamb	Loin, baby rack of lamb (trimmed of visible fat)
Game	Venison, buffalo, rabbit, caraboo, skinless duck breast, skinless pheasant, goose, ostrich

Dairy

As a rule, low-fat or skim milk dairy products and light or reduced-fat cheeses are used in the recipes. As in other animal proteins, full-fat dairy is actually higher in fat and saturated fat than meat. The only exceptions to using a low-fat cheese in the recipes in this book are those that use Parmesan. While moderately high in fat, Parmesan is a cheese that is used often because a little bit goes a long way for adding flavor to a dish, while not adding too much fat and calories. If you are watching your sodium intake because of medication or high blood pressure, aim to eat cheese that has 160 milligrams of sodium or less.

When cooking, it is tricky to find light or low-fat cheeses that taste good and that melt well. Below is a list of cheeses that I recommend because of their taste and composition. You can find most of them at your grocery store in the gourmet cheese section:

- Low-fat cheddar
- Low-fat havarti
- Lite jarlsburg
- Alpine Lace reduced-fat swiss
- Low-fat feta
- Low-fat goat cheese

- Light Boursin cheese (soft spread)
- Alouette light gourmet cheese (soft spread)
- Low-fat mozzerella
- Soy cheeses

A Word about Organic

The standards are changing for organic and becoming more streamlined and regimented. Below is a list of the new organic labeling that is currently being enforced. While the benefits of eating organic are not clearly defined, if you are pregnant or simply interested in minimizing your exposure to pesticides and added hormones, organic foods are worth considering. Some of the products you may want to consider are milk, yogurt, and cheeses (because they will not have the bovine growth hormone), produce, dried fruits (that do not contain sulfur), beef, eggs, and poultry (because you will minimize your exposure to antibiotic-laced feed that was given to the animals). If you don't go organic with meat and poultry you can find hormone-free meats available widely in your grocery store.

Coach Tip

You can identify organic produce by the USDA label, which verifies that the product is grown without conventional pesticides or petroleum-based fertilizers and the animal products are free of antibiotics and growth hormones.

The USDA Organic Seal will mean a product is either 95 or 100 percent organic—made from organic ingredients.

NO SEAL
Made with organic ingredients—products that contain 70 percent organic ingredients.

Some organic ingredients—products that contain less than 70 percent organic ingredients.

OTHER CLAIMS
100% Natural: Food contains no chemical ingredients but is not organic.
NO GMOs: No genetically modified foods are used as ingredients.
Hormone free: Animals were not fed hormones.

Healthy Cooking Made Easy: What to Have on Hand

Healthy cooking can be much easier for you when you have a well-stocked pantry and the proper equipment on hand. Below is a list of basic equipment that can save you time.

- A set of professional knives. At a minimum, you should have a good chef knife and paring knife, with a knife sharpener.
- Nonstick pans, pots, and baking sheets. Most important are nonstick sauté pans, so you can reduce the amount of fat you are using in recipes without food sticking to your pan. Look for sauté pans and pots with a thick bottom, which is better at transferring heat evenly, and handles that won't burn in the oven. For nonstick you will want to look for either copper or stainless pots and pans that are anodized so that the nonstick material does not scratch off easily.
- Measuring tools: liquid measuring cup, dry measuring cup, measuring spoons.
- Food processor
- Blender
- George Forman Grill (or other electric grill that allows the fat to drip away from the food that is cooking, or a stovetop iron grill)
- Japanese rice cooker or vegetable steamer

- Parchment paper
- Assorted small tools: zester, vegetable peeler, grater, large strainer, kitchen shears, large and small wire whisks, rubber spatulas and wooden spoons, meat mallet, tongs, spatulas for use with nonstick pots, slotted spoons, large spoons, soup ladle
- Timer
- Spray bottles for oil
- Storage containers for herbs, grains, nuts, dried fruit, etc.
- Mixing bowls: small, medium, and large (stainless, glass & ceramic are better than plastic)

Having certain pantry items on hand always makes it easier to cook, because when you go to the store to purchase ingredients for a recipe, you will already have a base from which to start at home. This will make the shopping trip much faster. Here is a list of basic items to keep on hand in the pantry and refrigerator/freezer:

- Canned broths—vegetable, chicken, and beef
- Thickeners—cornstarch or arrowroot
- Dried herbs and spices—thyme, rosemary, herbs de Provence, bouquet garni, Italian seasoning, black pepper, salt, curry, red chili flakes, cinnamon, nutmeg, ginger
- Oils—canola oil, olive oil, and extra virgin olive oil
- Vinegars—balsamic and raspberry
- Flours—whole wheat, almond, and all purpose (nonbleached)
- Grains and rices—rolled oats, low-fat granola, whole-grain bread and whole-wheat tortillas (low-fat)
- Evaporated skim milk
- Cooking wines—sherry, marsala, white, red, and mirin
- Sweeteners—honey, 100% pure maple syrup, fructose, granulated sugar, brown sugar
- Unsulfured dried fruits—cranberries, apricots, currants, cherries, dates
- Baking soda and baking powder
- Cocoa powder

- Flavorings—pure vanilla extract
- Nuts and seeds—slivered almonds, walnuts, pecans, pine nuts, sunflower, sesame, flax meal
- Canned artichoke hearts, chickpeas (garbanzo beans), black beans and other beans of choice, and sliced jalapeno peppers
- Pasta: whole-wheat spaghetti, prebaked lasagna noodles, whole-wheat couscous
- Jarred tomato sauce, diced tomatoes
- Tomato salsa

For the refrigerator/freezer:

- Frozen fruits—blueberries, peaches, raspberries (organic if possible)
- Salad dressings—low-fat Italian, Caesar
- Preserves—apricot and all-fruit cherry jam
- Low-fat or fat-free organic vanilla and plain yogurt
- Condiments—Grey Poupon mustard, all-natural ketchup
- Frozen apple juice concentrate
- Milk—low-fat buttermilk and skim milk
- Eggs or egg substitutes

Cooking Techniques—Losing the Fat but Not the Flavor

Fats carry flavor in foods and contribute to mouth-feel, the sensation you have from the food when you are eating it. When cooking low-fat there are several simple techniques I use to make sure the flavor is enhanced and you have plenty of mouth-feel. The first technique I call flavor layering. By layering on a particular flavor or flavors with several ingredients, you can be assured that you will really taste that particular flavor. An example of flavor layering would be a recipe that has orange flavor in it. In order to enhance the orange flavor, orange juice, orange zest, and oranges are used.

Marinating foods before cooking them is another great way to add flavor. Marinating both infuses the food with flavor and the marinades also act as tenderizers.

The texture is enhanced by having different types of textures for your mouth to feel while you are eating. This can be accomplished by using a variety of ingredients—nuts, seeds, vegetables, fruits. The more variety in texture that you can sense, the less likely you will be to miss the fat that has been removed from the recipe.

How to Flavor with Herbs

Below is a chart for you to use as a reference when flavoring with herbs. It will give you some general guidelines. Fresh or dried herbs are an easy way to add flavor. The flavor and aroma of herbs comes from their essential oils, which diminish over time when exposed to light and air. When using dried herbs, buy small amounts because they are only meant to be kept for six months before you need to buy new ones.

When cooking with herbs, it is helpful to think of the herbs as falling into two categories: (1) strong, robust herbs that are hearty and (2) light, delicate herbs. If you are making a hearty dish, such as turkey meat loaf or chicken in mushroom sauce, you would use the hearty herbs of thyme and rosemary with that dish, and a light dish, such as roasted salmon or chicken breast calls for lighter herbs that can include parsley, tarragon, or chives, so that the flavor of the herb does not overpower the food it is with.

	FLAVORS	GOOD IN
Strong-Robust Herbs		
Bay	Savory, warm spice	Soups and stews
Marjoram	Bold, floral tone with mint and pepper	Often found in Italian seasoning on roasted meats, tomato sauce: good with beans and hearty vegetables
Rosemary	Bold, pine/lemon flavors	Use with grilled and roasted meats, root vegetables, Mediterranean dishes, soups, stews, potatoes *(continued)*

	FLAVORS	GOOD IN
Sage	Strong savory and earthy	Use with roasted meats, stews
Savory	Strong woodsy	Use with roasted meats
Thyme	Moderate strength, lemon, pine, and spice flavors	Great with meat, seafood, poultry, hearty vegetables, soups, sauces, and Mediterranean dishes

Light-Delicate Herbs

Basil	Warm fresh mint/citrus flavors	Great fresh or cooked with vegetables, fish, poultry, sauces, salads, used in Mediterranean and Asian cooking
Chervil	Delicate slight anise/parsley flavor	Good garnish and complement to light fish, egg, or vegetable dishes
Chives	Mild onion flavor	Provides a great way to add a hint of onion to fish, chicken, and vegetables
Cilantro	Parsley/citrus flavor	A good, fresh-tasting complement to Asian, Spanish, and Indian cuisines: a natural with lime and chile
Dill	Warm green flavor	Pair with lighter meats, fish, seafood, eggs, and soups
Mint	Cool and fresh	Great with lamb, fruit, and desserts
Parsley	Fresh green flavor	Goes with almost anything: great as a garnish for soups, fish, vegetables, and chicken salads
Tarragon	Sweet with a slight licorice flavor	Works well with chicken, fish, eggs, seafood, and vegetables

Low-Fat Cooking Methods and Terms

Making low-fat foods is easy when you learn a few of the simple cooking methods that work to cut fat. Below is a chart of terms for you to know. When you absorb these cooking skills, you will be able to create your own quick meals using the same techniques.

Cooking Terms to Know

basting: To coat food with a liquid while it is cooking to moisten and prevent the surface from drying as it cooks.

blanching: To plunge food into rapidly boiling water and cook until softened or wilted. When done, plunge into cold water to stop the cooking process.

bouquet garni: A small bundle of aromatic herbs tied together in cheesecloth. A basic garni consists of several fresh parsley stems, a pinch of dried thyme, and a large bay leaf (or two small ones).

braising: To brown or sear over medium heat in a skillet on top of the stove. Then to add a bit of liquid—broth, water, juice or wine—and simmer over low heat until done.

broiling: A broiler heats from above. It is like an indoor grill, but a grill emits heat from below. The oven door is kept open slightly.

caramelize: To heat sugar or foods containing sugar (fruits) until the sugars in the food brown and develop a distinctive cooked flavor.

dry measure: A measuring cup that is only used to measure dry ingredients, where 1 cup equals 16 level tablespoons.

fold: To combine using two motions, one that cuts vertically through the mixture and the other that cuts horizontally. Often done gently so as not to disturb mixture or foam.

grilling: Use of heat from below to cook the food. The grill rack is coated with oil to prevent sticking.

(continued)

knife cuts:
- **chop**: Using quick, heavy knife cuts to cut food into bite-size pieces. A food processor may also be used to "chop" food.
- **cube**: Cut into ½-inch squares or cubes.
- **dice**: Cut into ¼-inch cubes.
- **mince**: Cut food into very small pieces (smaller than chopped food).
- **slice**: Cut food in long, thin slices.

liquid measure: Measuring tool with a capacity of one quart or less, and equipped with a lip for pouring. Often made of clear plastic or glass.

poach: To cook in a hot liquid.

puree: Blending a food until it is a liquid consistency.

roast: To cook by hot air in an oven with the door closed.

sauté: To brown or cook on the stovetop in a sauté pan that is lightly oiled.

sear: To brown the surface of meat or poultry in a sauté pan with intense heat applied for a short period of time.

simmer: To cook a liquid at a temperature that is just below boiling, 185 degrees.

sweat: Cook in a sauté pan in a small amount of spray oil or liquid (broth, wine, juice) over a medium flame until food is soft and begins to cook.

Key to the Recipes

As you plan your meals with *Gayle's Feel-Good Foods*, use the key on page 25 to determine which recipes fit in with the needs for your lifestyle or special occasions. Eating healthy every day can be quick and easy if you follow my easy shortcuts and recipes.

Recipe Icon Key

Quick and Easy

Ladies Luncheon

Kid-Friendly

Brunch

Make Ahead

Reduced Sugar

Elegant for Entertaining

Lower Sodium

Outdoor Grilling or Dining

2

Breakfast

Breakfast is a great Feel-Good way to start your day. Literally, breakfast breaks the fast from the evening and is the meal that revs up your body's engine—your metabolism—to burn food efficiently throughout the day. Recent research has actually shown that you can lose more weight by having breakfast than by skipping this meal.

Breakfast happens to be my favorite meal, because I love waking up and then indulging in delicious foods. I have included recipes here that are great to use any time. Some can be prepared ahead so you can enjoy a delicious homemade treat in the A.M., even if you are on the go. Others are a bit more elaborate, but breakfast food in general never takes that long to cook. So, if you have never made pancakes from scratch, give it a try: You will be surprised how easy it is.

Almond Oatmeal Pancakes

These pancakes are a delicious treat! The dry ingredients can be made ahead and stored in an airtight container.

YIELD: 14 PANCAKES

½ cup oat flour

¼ cup all-purpose flour

¼ cup finely ground almonds or almond flour

2 tablespoons honey

½ teaspoon salt

⅛ teaspoon nutmeg

⅛ teaspoon cinnamon

1 teaspoon baking soda

1¼ cups low-fat buttermilk

1 egg

½ teaspoon almond extract

Zest of one orange, grated

Oil for coating

1. Combine the flours, almonds, honey, salt, nutmeg, cinnamon, and baking soda. Mix with a fork.
2. In another bowl, whisk together the buttermilk, egg, almond extract, and zest. Pour the wet mixture into the flour mixture and gently stir to combine.
3. Heat a skillet on low-medium heat. Coat lightly with oil or spray with oil.
4. Drop the batter, ¼ cup at a time, onto the griddle, leaving space between pancakes for spreading.
5. Cook about 3 to 4 minutes, until you see bubbles on top of the pancakes. Flip and cook 2 more minutes.
6. Keep warm on a plate in the oven set at 200 degrees until all the pancakes are cooked.

Nutrition Facts:

Serving size 2 *pancakes,* Calories 100, *Fat* 2g, *Saturated Fat* 5g, *Cholesterol* 0mg, *Protein* 3g, *Carbohydrate* 16g, *Sugars* 7g, *Dietary Fiber* 1g, *Sodium* 394mg

Gayle's Feel-Good Facts

When you combine nuts with grains, it helps your blood sugar levels stay more balanced, so you are satiated for a longer period. This is because nuts are a heathy fat, and fats take longer to digest than grains or proteins.

Apple Butter

This is a great spread for bread that is low in sugar. As a sweetener, honey and dried fruit have been used. When you use this instead of butter or oil-based spreads you save on fat and feed your body protective nutrients. This spread keeps at least a month when stored in a sealed jar or container and refrigerated.

YIELD: 1 CUP

- 1 pound Granny Smith apples (approximately 3 apples), peeled and cored
- ¾ cup apple cider
- 3 tablespoons honey
- 1 teaspoon cinnamon
- ¼ teaspoon cloves
- ¼ teaspoon allspice
- ¼ teaspoon ginger
- ¼ cup date paste (found in produce section of grocery store), optional

1. Cut the apples into pieces. Put them in a pot, cover with the cider, honey, cinnamon, cloves, allspice, ginger, and date paste, and cook until soft, about 20 minutes.
2. Puree in a blender or food processor. Place the apple mixture back into the pot and cook over low heat until thick and smooth, stirring to prevent burning. You can test the thickness by placing a bit on a cold plate to see how solid it becomes.

Nutrition Facts:

Serving Size 3 tablespoons, *Calories* 110, *Fat* 0g, *Saturated Fat* 0g, *Cholesterol* 0mg, *Protein* 0g, *Carbohydrate* 30g, *Sugars* 22g, *Dietary Fiber* 3g, *Sodium* 0mg

Quick Tips for Making Breakfast

For baked goods, pancakes, and waffles: You can mix the dry mixture (flours, salts, seasonings, etc.) together and keep stored in a sealed container until needed. When ready to use, just add the wet mixture to the dry and cook. Breakfast breads and muffins can also be made ahead, frozen in portions, and reheated.

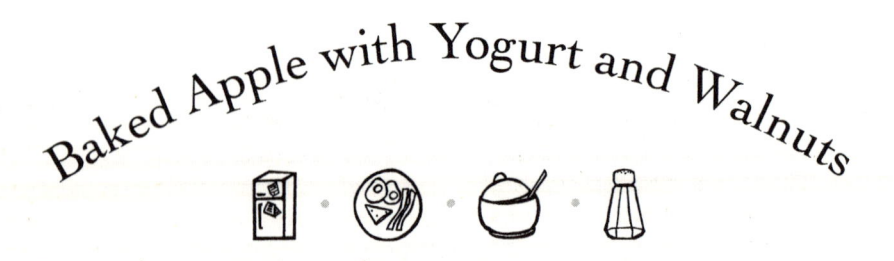

Baked Apple with Yogurt and Walnuts

This simple recipe can be made ahead and reheated or eaten cold. Warm apples are comforting and a great Feel-Good way to start the day.

YIELD: 4 SERVINGS

4 medium Rome apples, cored with ¾ inch opening (do not cut through to the bottom)

¼ cup apple juice or cider

Juice of one orange

½ cup water

2 tablespoons honey

4 tablespoons dried cranberries

4 tablespoons low-fat granola

4 teaspoons walnuts, chopped

Zest from 1 orange

1 cup vanilla nonfat yogurt

1. Preheat the oven to 375 degrees.
2. Peel the top half of each apple. Arrange the apples in a large, deep baking dish. Combine the apple juice or cider, orange juice, water, and 1 tablespoon of the honey in a small bowl. Pour into the baking dish up to ¼ inch deep. Cover tightly with a lid or foil and bake at 350 degrees until tender, about 40 minutes. Remove from the oven.
3. While the apples are baking, mix the remaining tablespoon of honey, the cranberries, granola, walnuts, zest, and yogurt in a medium mixing bowl, and set aside.
4. While the apples are still warm, fill with equal parts of the yogurt mixture and serve.

Nutrition Facts:

Serving Size 1 apple, *Calories* 240, *Fat* 25g, *Saturated Fat* 0g, *Cholesterol* 0mg, *Protein* 4g, *Carbohydrate* 54g, *Sugars* 44g, *Dietary Fiber* 5g, *Sodium* 50mg

Gayle's Feel-Good Fact

An apple a day actually can help prevent disease. Recent research at Cornell University showed that the natural plant compounds found in fruits are more protective than the vitamins by themselves. Other fruits where this holds true include blueberries, grapes, oranges, cranberries, and bananas.

Banana Bread

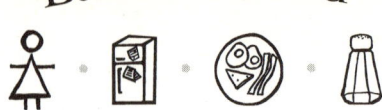

This bread is tasty but not too sweet, so it will satisfy you without triggering sweet cravings. The more ripe the bananas, the sweeter your bread will be. If you prefer muffins, you can use the same batter for a muffin tray of twelve.

YIELD: 12 SLICES OR 12 MUFFINS

1 large egg

¼ cup honey

½ cup fructose

1 cup smashed ripe bananas (about 3 medium)

⅓ cup low-fat buttermilk

2½ tablespoons canola oil

2 teaspoons vanilla extract

1 cup whole-wheat flour

¾ cup all-purpose flour

2 teaspoons baking powder

½ teaspoon baking soda

½ teaspoon salt

¼ cup carob chips, mini chocolate chips, or fruit juice–sweetened chocolate chips (these are available at most health food stores), optional

1. Preheat the oven to 325 degrees.
2. Lightly grease a 7½-x-3¾-x-2¼ non-stick loaf pan.
3. Using an electric mixer, beat the egg, honey, and fructose in a large bowl until thick and light, about 5 minutes. Mix in the smashed bananas, buttermilk, oil, and vanilla.
4. In a separate bowl, sift together flours, baking powder, baking soda, and salt. Add the wet mixture to the dry mixture and beat until just blended. Fold in the carob or chocolate chips, if using. Transfer the batter to prepared pan.
5. Bake the bread until golden brown on top and a tester inserted into the center comes out clean, about 1 hour. Turn the bread out onto a rack and cool.

Nutrition Facts:

Serving Size 1 slice or 1 muffin, *Calories* 170, *Fat* 3g, *Saturated Fat* 0g, *Cholesterol* 18mg, *Protein* 3g, *Carbohydrate* 33g, *Sugars* 17g, *Dietary Fiber* 3g, *Sodium* 121mg

If you use semi-sweet chocolate chips they add the following.
Calories 23, *Fat* 1g, *Saturated Fat* 1g, *Cholesterol* 0mg, *Protein* 0g, *Carbohydrate* 3g, *Sugar* 2g, *Dietary Fiber* 0g, *Sodium* 0mg

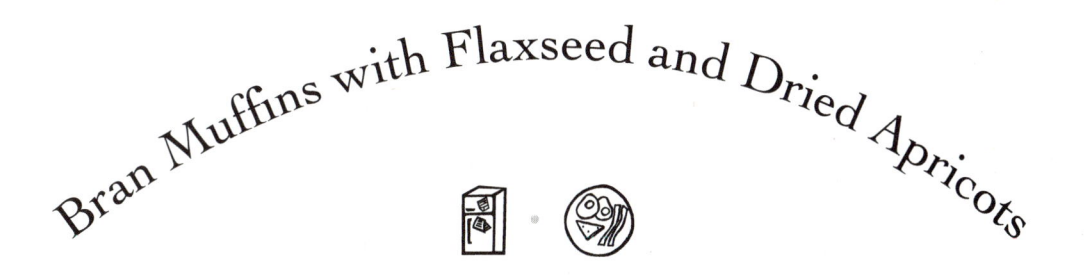

Bran Muffins with Flaxseed and Dried Apricots

This is a dense, hearty muffin with lots of flavor! Plus, the flaxseeds help you get your Omega-3 fats for the day.

YIELD: 12 MUFFINS

¾ cup whole-wheat flour	⅓ cup currants
¾ cup all-purpose unbleached white flour	1 cup chopped dried apricots
1 tablespoon baking powder	1 egg
2 teaspoons cinnamon	1⅓ cup low-fat buttermilk
¼ teaspoon grated nutmeg	2 tablespoons honey
⅓ cup brown sugar	2 teaspoon vanilla extract
1¼ cup bran cereal, such as Kellogg's All-Bran	3 tablespoons flaxseed

1. Preheat the oven to 400 degrees. Line a 12-compartment muffin tin with aluminum foil wrappers.

2. Put the flours, baking powder, cinnamon, nutmeg, brown sugar, bran cereal, currants, and apricots into a medium mixing bowl.
3. Put the egg, buttermilk, honey, and vanilla into another mixing bowl.
4. Mix the wet ingredients into the dry ingredients and fill the muffin tins ¾ full. Fold in the flaxseeds.
5. Bake for about 15 minutes, until cooked through. Enjoy.

Nutrition Facts:

Serving Size 1 muffin, *Calories* 161, *Fat* 2g, *Saturated Fat* .5g, *Cholesterol* 19mg, *Protein* 5g, *Carbohydrate* 33g, *Sugars* 15g, *Dietary Fiber* 4g, *Sodium* 15g

Breakfast Burritos

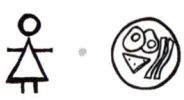

This is a tasty and fun way to eat eggs and vegetables in the A.M. Children will like this recipe, too.

YIELD: 4 SERVINGS

4 low-fat whole-wheat tortillas

½ cup chopped scallions

1 cup baby spinach leaves

½ cup tomato salsa

1 4-ounce can chopped green chilies, drained

2 large eggs

2 large egg whites

¼ cup grated low-fat cheddar

½ avocado, sliced

1. Heat the tortillas in a nonstick 8 or 12 inch skillet until warm. Keep warm in a 200 degree oven on parchment paper.

2. In a large nonstick skillet, add ⅓ of the scallions, baby spinach leaves, tomato salsa, and chilies. Cook until well blended, about 3 minutes on medium heat.
3. In a separate bowl mix together the eggs and egg whites until well blended, using a whisk or fork.
4. Pour the egg mixture into the pan and mix together with the vegetables until well blended and cook.
5. Place the egg mixture into the tortilla, sprinkle with cheddar and avocado slices.
6. Fold in the sides of the tortilla and roll from the bottom until the burrito is formed.
7. Serve warm. Can be kept warm in the 200-degree oven.

Nutrition Facts:

Serving Size 1 burrito, *Calories* 168, *Fat* 5g, *Saturated Fat* 1.5g, *Cholesterol* 107mg, *Protein* 11g, *Carbohydrate* 26g, *Sugars* 1g, *Dietary Fiber* 4g, *Sodium* 533mg

Quick Tip

You can buy the prewashed baby spinach and it will help you save time, because you won't have to cut the leaves. But be sure to rinse it again as it might have acquired some bacteria from sitting in the bag, even if it is prewashed.

Gayle's Feel-Good Facts

Whole eggs contribute some saturated fat to your diet, which can raise your cholesterol. If you are concerned about elevated cholesterol, substitute two egg whites for one egg or use egg substitute equivalent to the number of eggs in the recipe. The saturated fat and cholesterol are only in the yolk of the egg.

Gingerbread Pancakes

There is nothing that brings back memories of the holidays like the smell of gingerbread. These pancakes provide a comforting breakfast any time of the year.

YIELD: 7 SERVINGS

1¼ cups all-purpose flour	1 egg
1¼ cups whole-wheat flour	1 egg white
½ teaspoon baking powder	2 tablespoons apple juice concentrate
1 teaspoon baking soda	¼ cup firmly packed brown sugar
⅛ teaspoon salt	¾ cup low-fat buttermilk
2 teaspoons ground cinnamon	¼ cup water
2 teaspoons ground ginger	1 teaspoon butter
½ teaspoon ground nutmeg	2 teaspoons canola oil
⅛ teaspoon ground cloves	Oil spray
⅛ teaspoon allspice	

1. Combine the flours, baking powder, baking soda, salt, cinnamon, ginger, nutmeg, cloves, allspice, and brown sugar. Mix well and set aside.
2. In a separate bowl, combine the eggs, apple juice concentrate, and brown sugar, beating well.
3. Add the buttermilk, water, and butter; mix well.
4. Add the buttermilk mix to the dry ingredients, stirring just until moistened (batter will be slightly lumpy).
5. Grease a non-stick griddle or skillet with oil spray and set on low-medium heat. For each pancake, pour about ¼ cup of the batter onto the hot, greased griddle or skillet. Turn the pancakes when the tops are covered with bubbles and the edges are slightly dry.
6. Serve with apple butter (see page 29) and maple syrup, if desired.

Nutrition Facts:

Serving Size 2 pancakes, *Calories* 208, *Fat* 3g, *Saturated Fat* 1g, *Cholesterol* 34mg, *Protein* 8g, *Carbohydrate* 37g, *Sugars* 4g, *Dietary Fiber* 4g, *Sodium* 286mg

Gayle's Feel-Good Facts

Ginger is a spice that gives you a warming, stimulant effect on circulation, according to Asian philosophy, and it aids digestion.

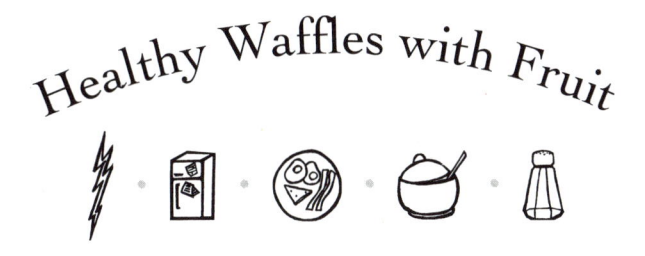

Healthy Waffles with Fruit

Waffles are a treat anytime. The fruit adds interesting texture and flavor, so don't hesitate to add your favorite fruits to the recipe. Below are some fruit suggestions. Waffles are also great to freeze, and keep for about a month in a sealed airtight freezer bag.

YIELD: 4 8-INCH WAFFLES

½ cup whole-wheat flour
½ cup all-purpose flour
1 teaspoon baking powder
½ teaspoon salt
¼ teaspoon baking soda

1 teaspoon cinnamon
½ cup fat free vanilla yogurt
½ cup skim milk
1 large egg yolk
2 teaspoons vanilla extract

2 tablespoons sugar
1 tablespoon canola oil
2 tablespoons honey

2 large egg whites
Oil spray

1. Preheat a waffle iron.
2. Mix together flours, baking powder, salt, baking soda, and cinnamon.
3. In a separate bowl mix the yogurt, skim milk, egg yolk, vanilla, canola oil, and honey.
4. Beat the egg whites until stiff. Add the sugar and continue beating until shiny. Fold a quarter of the beaten egg whites into the batter with a rubber spatula until well blended, then combine the remaining egg whites.
5. Spray the hot iron with oil. Fill an 8-inch wide iron with two-thirds cup of waffle batter. If the waffle iron is smaller, start with one-third cup of batter and add more if necessary to cover the iron. Cook for 4 to 6 minutes on medium until the waffles are cooked, a little longer for crisp waffles.

For Blueberry or Raspberry Waffles

Use 1 cup of fresh or frozen raspberries and sprinkle a quarter cup of the berries on the waffle batter prior to closing the iron.

For Strawberry or Banana Waffles

Use 1 cup of sliced strawberries or 2 bananas. Slice the fruit in 1/8-inch slices. For bananas, cut them in half and then slice the bananas. Sprinkle a quarter cup of the fruit on the waffle batter prior to closing the iron for cooking.

Nutrition Facts: For waffles with berries

Serving Size 1 waffle, *Calories* 227, *Fat* 3g, *Saturated Fat* 0g, *Cholesterol* 54mg, *Protein* 9g, *Carbohydrate* 39g, *Sugars* 16g, *Dietary Fiber* 2g, *Sodium* 417mg

Nutrition Facts: For waffles with strawberries

Calories 248, *Fat* 3gm, *Saturated Fat* 0g, *Cholesterol* 54mg, *Protein* 9g, *Carbohydrate* 44g, *Sugars* 19g, *Dietary Fiber* 3g, *Sodium* 417mg

Nutritional Facts: For waffles with bananas

Calories 254, *Fat* 3g, *Saturated Fat* 0g, *Cholesterol* 54mg, *Protein* 9g, *Carbohydrate* 46g, *Sugars* 21g, *Dietary Fiber* 3g, *Sodium* 417mg

Gayle's Feel-Good Facts

Berries are very low in calories, packed with protective nutrients including Vitamin C, and low on the glycemic index, so they don't raise your blood sugar as much as other fruits can. When your blood sugar is raised it stimulates you to eat more food. This can be a challenge if you are watching your portions in an effort to reduce calories and lose weight.

Low-Fat Chive Cream Cheese Spread

Use on whole-grain bread or crackers instead of butter. This healthy spread can be stored in the refrigerator for up to a week.

YIELD: 16 SERVINGS

½ pound low-fat cream cheese, room temperature

½ cup evaporated skim milk or nonfat plain yogurt

½ cup fresh chives, chopped

¼ cup fresh parsley (optional)

Pepper to taste

1. Place the cream cheese in a mixing bowl or food processor and blend until light and fluffy.
2. Add the milk or yogurt slowly, until the mixture has a spreadable consistency.
3. Mix in the chives and parsley (if desired) and season with pepper. Serve on toast for breakfast.

Nutrition Facts:

Serving Size 1 *tablespoon (*1 *ounce), Calories* 50, *Fat* 3g, *Saturated Fat* 1g, *Cholesterol* 0mg, *Protein* 2g, *Carbohydrate* 2g, *Sugars* 2g, *Dietary Fiber* 0g, *Sodium* 53mg

Low-Fat Salmon Cream Cheese Spread

A feel-good way to add taste to whole-grain bread, this spread also provides you with protein from the salmon. This spread will keep up to 2 weeks in the refrigerator.

YIELD: 16 SERVINGS

½ *pound low-fat cream cheese, room temperature*

½ *cup evaporated skim milk or nonfat plain yogurt*

¼ *pound nova salmon, chopped*

Pepper to taste

1. Place the cream cheese in a mixing bowl or food processor and blend until light and fluffy.
2. Add the milk or yogurt slowly, until the mixture has a spreadable consistency.
3. Mix in the salmon. Season with pepper. Serve on toast for breakfast.

Nutrition Facts:

Serving Size 2 tablespoons (1 ounce), *Calories* 50, *Fat* 3g, *Saturated Fat* 2g, *Cholesterol* 10mg, *Protein* 3g, *Carbohydrate* 2g, *Sugars* 2g, *Dietary Fiber* 0g, *Sodium* 194mg

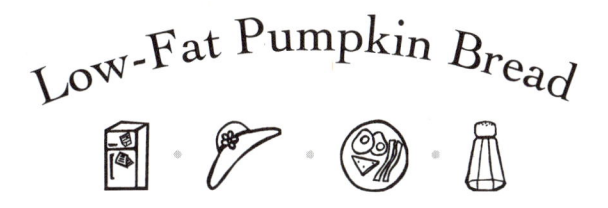

Low-Fat Pumpkin Bread

A perfect way to get into the fall spirit any time of year! Warm up a slice of bread as a breakfast treat. You can also use this same recipe for muffins.

YIELD: 14 SLICES OR 12 MUFFINS

2 egg whites

1 cup sugar

1 cup fat-free yogurt

2 tablespoons canola oil

1 cup grated carrot

3 cups pumpkin puree (fresh or canned)

2 tablespoons cinnamon

1 teaspoon ginger

½ teaspoon clove

½ teaspoon salt

3 cups all-purpose unbleached flour (can use ½ whole-wheat or whole-grain flour)

1 tablespoon baking soda

2 teaspoons baking powder

1. Preheat oven to 350 degrees.
2. In a large bowl combine the egg whites, sugar, yogurt, oil, carrots, and pumpkin puree. Mix well.
3. In a separate bowl combine the spices, flour, baking soda, and baking powder.
4. Mix the pumpkin mixture with the dry mixture. Stir just until well blended.
5. Pour the batter into a large non-stick loaf pan, that has been sprayed or lightly coated with oil.

6. Bake for 55 minutes. The bread is ready when the center is firm. Use a fork or skewer to insert in the middle of bread. If the bread is not firm, turn the oven down to 325 degrees and continue baking for 15 to 20 minutes. When cooked, allow the bread to cool to room temperature. If storing, remove bread onto a wire cooling rack and cool completely. Wrap with plastic wrap and store in the refrigerator or freeze. *Keep the bread stored in the refrigerator so it maintains its moisture.*

Nutrition Facts:

Serving Size 1 slice or 1 muffin, *Calories* 168, *Saturated Fat* 0g, *Cholesterol* 0mg, *Protein* 4g, *Carbohydrate* 35g, *Sugars* 16g, *Dietary Fiber* 2g, *Sodium* 266mg

Gayle's Feel-Good Facts

The orange color of pumpkin, like that of carrots, helps give away the fact that it is high in carotenes, an antioxidant that helps prevent cancer. For ease of use, feel free to opt for the canned pumpkin. It is just as nutritious as the fresh and a lot less work.

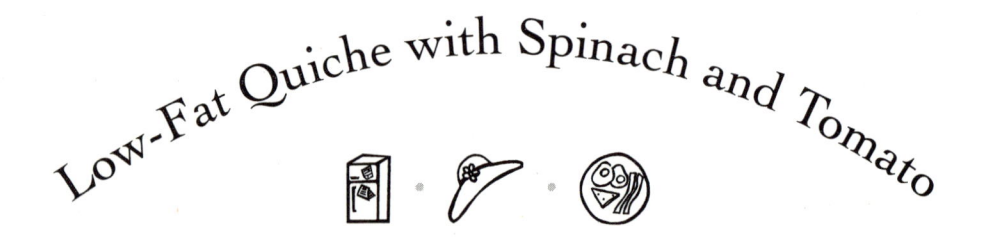

Low-Fat Quiche with Spinach and Tomato

This quiche wins rave reviews from all who eat it! A good breakfast item, or it can be used for lunch too!

YIELD: 10 SERVINGS

1 ready-made piecrust from freezer section of grocery store

1 cup skim milk

4 large egg whites

1/8 teaspoon salt (2 pinches)

⅛ teaspoon black pepper

⅛ teaspoon nutmeg

½ pound baby spinach

½ large onion, sliced

Oil spray

⅓ cup low-fat chedder

1 large tomato (or 2 small), sliced

1. Preheat the oven to 350 degrees.
2. Prick the piecrust with a fork to prevent bubbles in the crust. Precook the crust in a 350-degree oven for 7 minutes, until slightly browned. Set aside.
3. While the piecrust is baking, in a large bowl add the skim milk and egg whites. Stir gently to avoid too many bubbles. Add the salt, pepper, and nutmeg. Refrigerate until ready to use.
4. To cook the spinach, heat a nonstick sauté pan until warm. Place the rinsed spinach in the pan and let wilt on low-medium heat. If necessary, add a few drops of water to the pan to prevent the spinach from burning and be sure not to set the heat too high.
5. To cook the onions, spray sauté pan with oil spray. On medium heat sauté onions for about 4 minutes or until they are soft. If the onions begin to stick to the pan, add a tablespoon or two of water to the skillet to prevent the onions from burning.
6. Spread the sautéed onions on the bottom of the crust in a thin layer.
7. Sprinkle the cooked spinach on top of the onions. Then, add the shredded cheese. Ladle the egg mixture over the spinach. Make ¼ slices of tomato to lay on top of the quiche to decorate.
8. Bake for 35 to 40 minutes. If the crust edges are too dark, lightly cover the quiche with foil. When the center is not loose, the quiche is cooked. Remove from the oven and serve.

Nutrition Facts:

Serving Size 1 slice, *Calories* 97, *Fat* 3g, *Saturated Fat* 1g, *Cholesterol* 5mg, *Protein* 4g, *Carbohydrate* 11g, *Sugars* 2g, *Dietary Fiber* 0g, *Sodium* 184mg

Quick Tip

Using a piecrust from the store is the easiest way to go low-fat, because it is difficult to make a low-fat piecrust by hand that is easy to roll out or that achieves a flaky texture. I recommend the Pet Ritz or Orchards frozen piecrusts, because of their lower fat content. Although both piecrust recommendations are not made with whole grain, when you are looking for convenience, these piecrusts offer the best option. Also, it is difficult to make a low-fat whole-wheat or whole-grain crust, so here is where you can use the exception to the rule in order to stay low-fat and still eat piecrust.

Traditional Pancakes

These pancakes have a traditional flavor, but they are also packed with fiber from the whole-grain flour, oats, and flax meal. Once you have the ingredients in your house, these take no time to mix together.

YIELD: 8 SERVINGS

2 teaspoons canola oil

1¼ cups low-fat buttermilk

1 large egg

2 tablespoons honey

¼ cup whole-grain or whole-wheat flour

½ cup all-purpose flour

2 tablespoons flax meal

¾ cups rolled oats

1 teaspoon baking powder

½ teaspoon baking soda

½ teaspoon cinnamon

Pinch of salt

1. In a large mixing bowl, combine the oil, buttermilk, egg, and honey. Whisk together.
2. In a large bowl, combine the flours, flax meal, oats, baking powder, baking soda, cinnamon, and salt.
3. Make a well in the center of the dry mixture and gently pour the wet mixture into the dry mixture.
4. Stir to combine, but do not overbeat. Let sit for 15 to 20 minutes.
5. Spray a large griddle or frying pan with oil to coat. Heat on low-medium heat.
6. Once the pan is hot, drop ¼ cup of pancake batter at a time onto the griddle. Allow to cook about 3 minutes, until you see bubbles and the edges look cooked. Then flip and cook about 2 minutes more. If you make larger pancakes, increase the cooking time to an initial 4 to 5 minutes, then flip.
7. The pancakes can be kept warm in a 200-degree oven while you make the full batch.

Nutrition Facts:

Serving Size 2 pancakes, *Calories* 119, *Fat* 3g, *Saturated Fat* 0g, *Cholesterol* 29mg, *Protein* 6g, *Carbohydrate* 18g, *Sugars* 2g, *Dietary Fiber* 3g, *Sodium* 193mg

Adding Fruit to your Pancakes

Fruit on pancakes makes a colorful presentation. If you want to add fruit to your pancakes, the fruit will sink to the bottom if the batter is too thin. This batter works well, so feel free to add any fruit you would like and pack extra nutrition into every bite. Add the fruit to the dry mixture before you mix it with the wet mixture. Use 1 cup of chopped fruit per recipe.

Gayle's Feel-Good Facts

Jams or preserves that do not have added sugar make a great accompaniment to breads for an added burst of sweetness. Use sparingly, so they don't contribute too much sugar to your meal. A sugar high will cause you to feel tired later.

(continued)

If you like, you can blend your favorite jam with low-fat cream cheese, thereby cutting the sweetness and adding a light cheese flavor. Good flavors to try are cherry, peach, or berry preserves.

Gayle's Feel-Good Facts

Using maple syrup is fine on pancakes, but it can add up calorically, so use it sparingly. Two tablespoons is a good amount to aim for per serving of pancakes or waffles.

Classic Spanish Omelette

This is a low-fat version of a Spanish favorite. It is a more elegant way to serve an omelette and it can be cut into small slices like a pie for appetizers.

YIELD: 10 SERVINGS

2 tablespoons olive oil

1 large onion, sliced into 1/8-inch slices

1/2 teaspoon salt

2 eggs

4 egg whites

1. Heat half the oil in a 10-inch nonstick or well-seasoned skillet over medium heat.
2. Add the sliced onion and a ½ teaspoon of the salt. Cook until the onions are tender, about 10 minutes.
3. Beat the eggs with the egg whites in a bowl with the remaining ½ teaspoon of salt. Add the cooked onions to the eggs.
4. In the original skillet add the remaining oil and spread it around the pan. Add the egg mixture, shaking the pan to avoid sticking. Cook just until the eggs are set, about 5 minutes.
5. Cover the pan with a large plate or wide lid. Holding the lid firmly with the flat of your hand, turn the pan upside down. Slide the omelette from the plate or lid back into the pan on the noncooked side and cook for about 2 to 5 minutes. A skewer or fork inserted into the center should come out clean.
6. Spanish omelettes can be served hot, warm, or room temperature. Cut the omelette into wedges and serve. It can be a great lunch item as well.

▪ *Other Filling Combinations to Try*

Spinach and onion, Onions and mushrooms, Potato and onion, Cheese (low-fat feta, goat, or cheddar) and tomato, Peppers and onion.

Nutrition Facts for classic omelette:

Serving Size 1/10 slice, Calories 53, Fat 3g, Saturated Fat 0g, Cholesterol 43mg, Protein 3g, Carbohydrate 2g, Sugars 1g, Dietary Fiber 0g, Sodium 172mg

½ cup cheese adds the following nutrition (approximate values) per serving: Calories 16, Fat 1g, Saturated Fat 1g, Cholesterol 9mg, Protein 2g, Carbohydrate 0g, Sugars 0g, Dietary Fiber 0g, Sodium 14mg.

Nutrition Facts:

When adding cheese, omit a teaspoon of oil to keep the recipe low-fat.

Vegetables are so low in calories they are unlimited. When adding vegetables to the omelette, follow the procedures for the onions using your vegetable(s) of choice.

Zucchini Bread

The lemon and sunflower seeds add zest to this traditional loaf bread. Since the bread is not too sweet, you can have this alongside any meal—breakfast, lunch, or dinner.

YIELD: 1 LOAF (10 SLICES) OR 12 MUFFINS

3 medium zucchini, shredded (about 2 cups)	¼ cup grape juice concentrate
1 cup whole-wheat flour	¼ cup honey
1 cup all-purpose flour	½ cup vanilla soy milk
⅓ cup fructose	3 tablespoons canola oil
1 teaspoon baking powder	1 teaspoon vanilla extract
2 teaspoons baking soda	¼ cup applesauce, unsweetened
1 tablespoon lemon peel	1 egg
1 tablespoon cinnamon	½ cup currants
⅛ teaspoon salt	1 cup sunflower seed, dry roasted.
¼ teaspoon nutmeg	

1. Preheat the oven to 350 degrees.
2. Press the zucchini on several layers of paper towels. Cover with additional paper towels and set aside.
3. Combine the flours, ⅓ cup fructose, baking powder, baking soda, lemon peel, cinnamon, salt, and nutmeg in a large bowl; make a well in the center of the mixture.
4. In a separate bowl, combine the grape juice concentrate, honey, vanilla soy milk, oil, vanilla, applesauce, molasses, and egg; stir with a whisk. Add the zucchini; stir. Fold in the currants. Add to the flour mixture by placing in the well; stir just until moist.

5. Spray a (8x4-inch) loaf pan with cooking spray and pour in the batter. Sprinkle the sunflower seeds on top of the batter. If making muffins, fill a muffin pan for 12 muffins and sprinkle sunflower seeds evenly on all 12 muffins.
6. Bake the zucchini bread in the center of the oven until cooked through, about 1 hour. If making muffins, bake for 20 to 25 minutes. Bread or muffins are done when fork or cake tester comes out clean.

Nutrition Facts:
Serving Size 1 slice or 1 muffin, *Calories* 178, *Fat* 3g, *Saturated Fat* .5g, *Cholesterol* 18mg, *Protein* 4g, *Carbohydrate* 33g, *Sugars* 12g, *Dietary Fiber* 3g, *Sodium* 266mg

Gayle's Feel-Good Facts

Sunflower seeds are packed with omega-6 essential fats, as well as vitamin E, an antioxidant that helps prevent against heart disease, cancers, and cataracts. When cooked, the vitamin E is retained.

3

Appetizers and Party Foods

In my opinion, good food helps make a party special, so in this section I have put together some of my favorite recipes for healthy finger foods that by no means taste healthy. If you are watching your weight or your fat intake, finding recipes to serve at parties is typically very difficult. But now you will not have to feel like you have to watch what you are eating since all the recipes in this section are healthy and guilt-free. Your guests will not know the difference, whether what you are serving is healthy or not, so it is your choice if you want to divulge your secret. But, with so many people watching what they eat, I would think your guests will be pleasantly surprised at how good low-fat party food can be. If you are planning to have a large party and use a caterer, you can pass on some of these recipes to the chef, so you don't have to feel compromised if healthy fare is your preference. Enjoy the party and have fun indulging!

Lite Cheese Fondue

Fondues offer a tasty way to serve vegetables at a party. It is best to use a fondue pot, but if you don't have one, you can make this sauce in a heavy saucepan and then cover the vegetables in the sauce instead of dipping them.

YIELD: 14 SERVINGS

1 clove garlic

1 cup plus 2 tablespoons dry white wine

1 teaspoon lemon juice, fresh squeezed

1 tablespoon brandy or vodka

1 tablespoon cornstarch

7 ounces lite Jarlsburg, grated

7 ounces low-fat cheddar, grated

½ teaspoon salt

Ground fresh black pepper to taste

1. Slice the garlic clove in half and rub the garlic pieces around the inside of the fondue pot.
2. Add the wine and lemon juice and gently warm in the fondue pot over the fondue flame.
3. Mix the brandy or vodka with the cornstarch, set aside.
4. Stir the cheeses into the fondue pot and keep stirring to prevent sticking until melted. Do not let the mixture boil.
5. When cheese is melted add the cornstarch mixture and continue stirring until the cheese mixture becomes thick. Season with salt and pepper.
6. Serve fondue with cubes of whole-grain bread, grape tomatoes, and steamed vegetables.

Nutrition Facts:

Serving Size 1 ounce, Calories 67, Fat 3g, Saturated Fat 1g, Cholesterol 6mg, Protein 7g, Carbohydrate 1g, Sugars 0g, Dietary Fiber 0g, Sodium 257mg

> Phyllo dough is a great dough to work with when you are cooking low-fat. However, it is paper thin, so taking precautions to prevent it from drying out while you are using it is essential. You can purchase a one-pound package of phyllo dough in the freezer section of the grocery store. When you are ready to use it, allow it to thaw in the refrigerator for one to two days. Or follow the directions on the package and let it defrost outside of the refrigerator.
>
> When you are ready to use it, unwrap it from its package and lay the leaves on plastic wrap on the counter. Cover the top of the dough with a slightly damp cloth to prevent it from drying out.

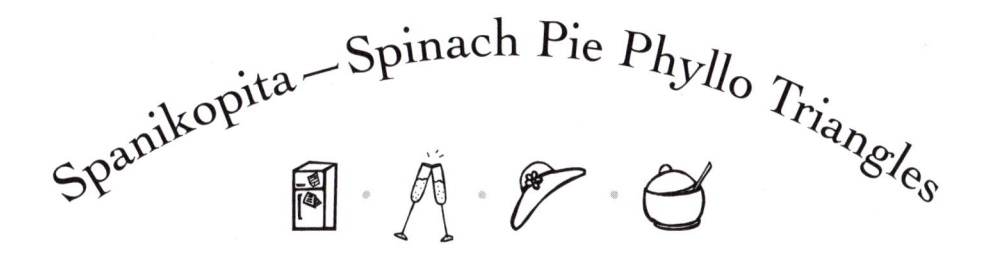

Spanikopita—Spinach Pie Phyllo Triangles

This traditional Greek appetizer offers a great pastry-filled starter or hors d'oeuvres without all the butter (saturated fat) that is typically found in dough-filled appetizers.

YIELD: 18 TO 20 SERVINGS

- 10 ounces frozen chopped spinach, defrosted
- ½ yellow onion, finely chopped
- 1 tablespoon extra virgin olive oil
- ⅓ cup crumbled reduced fat feta cheese
- ¼ cup low-fat or part skim ricotta
- ½ cup chopped dill
- ¼ teaspoon nutmeg
- ¼ teaspoon garlic powder
- ¼ teaspoon salt
- ½ teaspoon black pepper
- 1 pound phyllo dough, thawed (found in freezer section of grocery store)
- Oil spray

1. Preheat the oven to 350 degrees.
2. Drain the defrosted spinach of all excess water by placing it in a strainer and forcing the water out by squeezing down the spinach with your hand or a large spoon.
3. In a large mixing bowl, combine all the spinach, onion, olive oil, feta, ricotta, dill, nutmeg, garlic, salt, and pepper and mix well. Set aside.
4. Peel one sheet of dough from the pack. Place on a flat work surface, spray with oil spray, and then repeat until you have 3 sheets of dough stacked together. Using a sharp knife, cut the dough into 5 equal strips along the shorter side of the dough.
5. To fill, place one teaspoon of filling on the end nearest you. Fold over diagonally, so the right corner of the dough meets the other side. Continue folding the dough packet over itself so that it forms a triangular-shaped pie. Spray the top with oil spray and place on a nonstick or foil-lined cookie sheet. Repeat folding procedure with remaining dough and spinach filling.
6. Bake until cooked through and light brown, approximately 25 minutes. Serve warm.

Nutrition Facts:

Serving Size 1 triangle, *Calories* 73, *Fat* 2g, *Saturated Fat* 6g, *Cholesterol* 2mg, *Protein* 3g, *Carbohydrate* 10g, *Sugars* 0g, *Dietary Fiber* 2g, *Sodium* 160mg

Quick Tip

This appetizer or healthy snack can be made ahead, frozen, and reheated a few at a time. To reheat from frozen, place frozen Spanikopita on a nonstick or foil-lined baking sheet. Bake in 350 degree oven for 35 to 45 minutes, until well heated and slightly browned.

Artichoke Dip

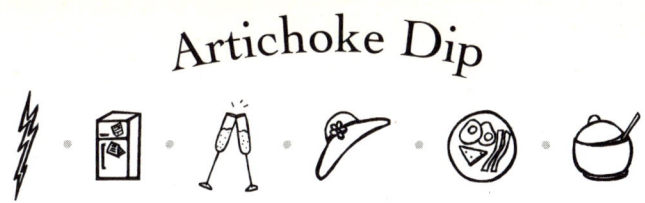

This traditional Italian spread makes an excellent party starter with vegetables and crackers.

YIELD: 2 CUPS (16 SERVINGS)

1 14-ounce can artichoke hearts, drained

2 tablespoons extra virgin olive oil

¼ cup Parmesan cheese, grated

Juice of ½ lemon

1. Combine all the ingredients in a blender or food processor and puree until well blended.
2. Serve with breadsticks or cut cucumber, carrots, and/or red peppers.

Nutrition Facts:

Serving Size 1 tablespoon, *Calories* 32, *Fat* 2g, *Saturated Fat* 0g, *Cholesterol* 1mg, *Protein* 1.5g, *Carbohydrate* 3g, *Sugars* 0g, *Dietary Fiber* 1g, *Sodium* 53mg

Roasted Red Pepper Aioli

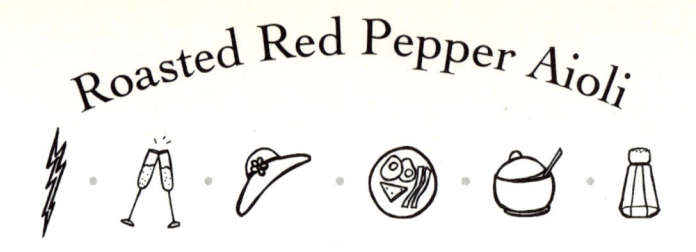

Great as a dip or spread for sandwiches.

YIELD: 4 SERVINGS

1 red pepper
2 tablespoons low-fat mayo
Pinch of salt and pepper

1. Place the pepper on a baking sheet and roast in a 450-degree oven until all sides are black and charred. Take out of the oven and cover with a paper bag or plastic wrap. When cool, peel the skin off the pepper by rubbing the outside with a paper towel.
2. In a blender or food processor, place the red pepper and low-fat mayo. Puree.
3. Season with salt and pepper. Store in an airtight container in the refrigerator.

Nutrition Facts:

Serving Size 2 *tablespoons, Calories* 20, *Fat* 0g, *Saturated Fat* 0g, *Cholesterol* 0mg, *Protein* 0g, *Carbohydrate* 3g, *Sugars* 2g, *Dietary Fiber* 0g, *Sodium* 143mg

Gayle's Feel-Good Facts

When you use vegetables as a base for dips you save on many calories, plus it is an easy way to take in the protective nutrients from vegetables. The American Cancer Society recommends we eat nine fruits and vegetables a day.

Avocado Tomatillo Salsa

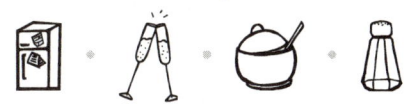

A party favorite and great item to put out for your guests.

YIELD: 16 SERVINGS (2 TABLESPOONS)

8 ounces tomatillos (about 5 tomatillos) fresh, seeded, steamed

1 ounce canned jalapenos (approximately 2 peppers) chopped

½ cup chopped cilantro

3 ounces chopped white onions (1 onion)

2 garlic cloves, peeled

¼ cup chicken broth or vegetable broth

1½ avocados, diced

¼ teaspoon salt

1. Blend tomatillos, jalapenos, cilantro, onion, garlic, and chicken or vegetable broth until smooth.
2. Add the avocados and salt to the blended mixture.
3. Serve with baked tortilla chips, which are easily found at your local supermarket or health food store.

Nutrition Facts:

Serving Size 2 tablespoons, *Calories* 53, *Fat* 3g, *Saturated Fat* 1g, *Cholesterol* 0mg, *Protein* 1g, *Carbohydrate* 3g, *Sugars* 0g, *Dietary Fiber* 1g, *Sodium* 99mg

Gayle's Feel-Good Facts

While most people think avocado is fattening (with a negative connotation), the truth is avocado is very healthy. It is a good fat, loaded with the beneficial omega-3 fats. It is important to watch your portions when you eat avocado, because it is high in calories, but it is good for you. So, don't avoid it.

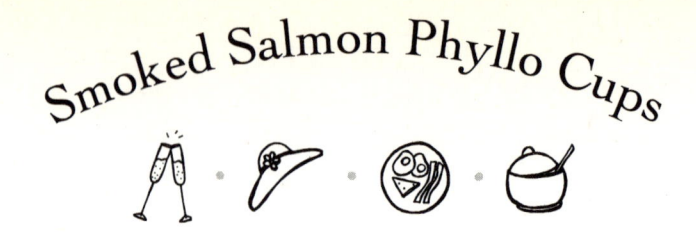

Smoked Salmon Phyllo Cups
with Herbed Cheese Spread

A favorite from my catering days, these fancy little tarts are both tasty and attractive. A hit with any gathering!

YIELD: 12 SERVINGS

- 12 mini phyllo tart or canapé shells
- 4 ounces low-fat goat cheese
- 1 cup fat-free ricotta
- 12 ounces fat-free cream cheese
- ½ teaspoon salt
- ½ teaspoon pepper
- 1 teaspoon lemon juice
- ¼ cup chopped dill
- ¼ pound smoked Norwegian salmon, sliced
- 4 sprigs fresh dill, cut into ½-inch pieces

1. Preheat the oven to 350 degrees. If using frozen phyllo tart shells, take them out of the freezer and bake in the oven for 5 minutes on a baking sheet. Remove and let cool.
2. Combine the cheeses, salt, pepper, lemon juice, and dill in a food processor until smooth. Set aside in the refrigerator.
3. Slice the salmon into 1-inch strips and roll them up loosely from one end to the other.
4. Using a tablespoon, dollop one large tablespoon of cheese spread into each tart or canapé shell. Top with one of the salmon rolls, wide side down. Using your fingers, open up the salmon rolls a bit so they resemble a flower. Place a ½ piece of dill in the center of the roll as decoration.
5. Serve at room temperature.

Nutrition Facts:

Serving Size 1 tart, *Calories* 93, *Fat* 3g, *Saturated Fat* 1g, *Cholesterol* 7.5mg, *Protein* 11g, *Carbohydrate* 5g, *Sugars* 1g, *Dietary Fiber* 0g, *Sodium* 511mg

Hummus

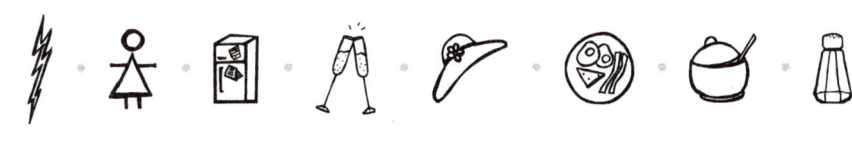

This is a low-fat favorite of a traditional Mediterranean dip.

YIELD: 8 SERVINGS

15-ounce can garbanzo beans

2 to 3 tablespoons lemon juice

2 tablespoons fresh parsley, chopped

¼ cup fat-free yogurt

1 teaspoon cumin

½ teaspoon allspice

1 large clove garlic, minced

Pinch of salt

Pinch of pepper

Pinch of cayenne, optional

2 tablespoons tahini sauce

1. Rinse and drain the garbanzo beans.
2. Combine all the ingredients in the food processor and puree until smooth.
3. Add a little water if the mixture is too thick.
4. Season with salt and pepper to taste.

Nutrition Facts:

Serving Size ¼ cup, *Calories* 106, *Fat* 3g, *Saturated Fat* 0g, *Cholesterol* 0mg, *Protein* 6g, *Carbohydrate* 16g, *Sugars* 1g, *Dietary Fiber* 4g, *Sodium* 46mg

Gayle's Feel-Good Facts

Bean dips make smart snacks because they are high in protein and low in calories and carbs, compared to most dips. Try them with cut-up vegetables, which will add fiber to your day and also keep you satiated longer.

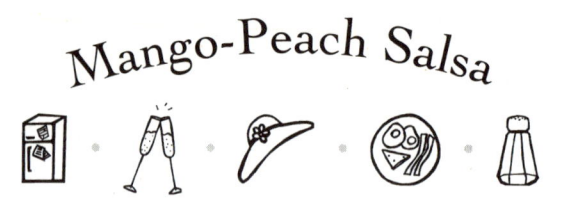

Mango-Peach Salsa

Salsas are usually a Mexican sauce that is composed of tomato, chilies, onion, and peppers. Using fruit as a base gives salsa a nice sweet taste. I like serving it at a party because it is colorful and the balance of the spicy and sweet is a nice combination. Serve with your favorite brand of baked tortilla chips, which you can purchase at the supermarket or health food store.

YIELD: 14 SERVINGS

- 2 mangos (about 1½ cups), diced
- 3 peaches (about 1½ cups), diced
- 2 red bell peppers, diced
- 1 small mild green chile, minced
- ¼ cup vegetable broth
- 2 tablespoons chopped cilantro
- 2 teaspoons white wine or champagne vinegar
- Dash of Tabasco, to taste
- ½ teaspoon fructose

1. Gently combine all the ingredients in a medium mixing bowl.
2. Cover and refrigerate until ready to serve.

Nutrition Facts:

Serving Size ¼ cup, Calories 20, Fat 0g, Saturated Fat 0g, Cholesterol 0mg, Protein 0g, Carbohydrate 5g, Sugars 6g, Dietary Fiber 1g, Sodium 36mg

Gayle's Feel-Good Facts

Mango can be considered a "power food" because it is high in most of the protective nutrients—vitamin E, vitamn C, and, like other orange fruits, the carotenes.

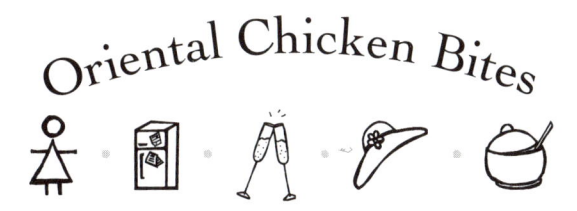

Oriental Chicken Bites

What a treat! These Asian chicken balls with almonds are a substantial starter or finger food. They can be served hot or room temperature, and they can be made ahead and frozen. I have never known them not to be a hit at a party.

YIELD: 40 PIECES

1¼ pound chicken breast

4½ tablespoons low-sodium soy sauce

4 tablespoons bread crumbs

½ teaspoon salt

½ teaspoon sesame oil (hot sesame oil if desired)

2 cloves garlic, minced

1-inch slice ginger, pressed, or 1/2-inch slice ginger minced

1 egg white

⅓ cup scallions, sliced thin

COATING

2 egg whites

10 ounces almonds, chopped

SAUCE

½ cup low-sodium soy sauce

¼ cup sherry

¼ teaspoon sesame oil

3 tablespoons honey

1 teaspoon peeled and finely chopped ginger

¼ teaspoon finely chopped medium garlic clove

¼ teaspoon lime juice

1. Grind the chicken in a food processor until well chopped. Add the low-sodium soy sauce, bread crumbs, salt, sesame oil, garlic, ginger, and egg white. Blend until well mixed. If not using a food processor, purchase ground chicken breast and mix in ingredients with a large mixing spoon in a large bowl until well blended.
2. Add the scallions at end and pulse 2 times.
3. Flour your hands and roll the chicken mixture in 1-inch balls. In a small bowl, whip up the egg to use as an egg wash. Dip the chicken balls into the egg wash and then dip in the almonds to coat each ball.
4. Bake for 10 to 15 minutes, until firm.
5. Mix all sauce ingredients in a medium bowl.
6. Serve chicken balls warm with dipping sauce on the side.

Nutrition Facts for Chicken Bites:

Serving Size 1 chicken ball, *Calories* 44, *Fat* 3g, *Saturated Fat* 0g, *Cholesterol* 9mg, *Protein* 5g, *Carbohydrate* 1g, *Sugars* 0g, *Dietary Fiber* 0g, *Sodium* 98mg

Nutrition Facts for Sauce:

Serving size ½ teaspoon, *Calories* 3, *Fat* 0g, *Saturated Fat* 0g, *Cholesterol* 110mg, *Protein* 0g, *Carbohydrate* 1g, *Sugars* 1g, *Dietary Fiber* 0g, *Sodium* 45mg

Quick Tip

Using flavored or infused oils (oils with added herbs) is an easy way to impart flavor to a low-fat dish, because the oil will carry the seasoning throughout the food, adding a pleasurable taste sensation to every bite.

Cajun Chicken Fingers

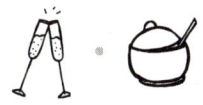

Tasty morsels that are sure to give your mouth a kick!

YIELD: 18 TO 20 PIECES

CHICKEN SPICE RUB

1 teaspoon black pepper

1 teaspoon garlic powder

2 teaspoons dry mustard

2½ teaspoons cayenne

2 teaspoons white pepper

1½ teaspoons ground sage

2 teaspoons salt

2 teaspoons ground thyme

CHICKEN

1 cup whole-grain or whole-wheat flour

2 egg whites

1¼ pounds chicken breast, cut in 1-inch strips

1 egg

CILANTRO SOUR CREAM

1 cup fat-free sour cream

2 dashes hot sauce, such as Tabasco (optional)

½ cup chopped cilantro

Juice of 1 lime (2 teaspoons)

1. Mix together all ingredients for spice rub into a large shallow container.
2. In a medium bowl, combine 3 tablespoons of the spice mixture with the flour. Reserve remaining spice rub for later use. Place the mixture in a shallow dish or plate in preparation to coat the chicken.
3. In a large shallow bowl, scramble the egg whites and set aside.

4. Dip each chicken strip first in the egg then in the flour mixture.
5. Spray a nonstick skillet with oil spray. Sear chicken on a medium-high flame 1 minute on each side until browned, then place on a baking tray and place in the oven at 350 degrees to finish cooking for 5 minutes. Turn oven off to keep chicken warm while you finish preparing the sauce.
6. Combine all cilantro sour cream ingredients in a medium bowl and refrigerate until ready to use.
7. Serve the chicken warm with cilantro sour cream for dipping.

Nutrition Facts:

Serving Size 1 piece (1 oz), *Calories* 82, *Fat* 2.5g, *Saturated Fat* 6g, *Cholesterol* 34mg, *Protein* 10g, *Carbohydrate* 4g, *Sugars* 0g, *Dietary Fiber* 1g, *Sodium* 75mg

Cilantro Sour Cream:

Serving Size 1 oz, *Calories* 15, *Fat* 0g, *Saturated Fat* 0g, *Cholesterol* 1mg, *Protein* 1g, *Carbohydrate* 3g, *Sugars* 1g, *Dietary Fiber* 0g, *Sodium* 13g.

Chicken Saté with Lite Peanut Sauce

Peanut sauce is always a favorite. Now you can have it guilt free with this lite version. It is always popular at any party or celebration. It is quick to make and will win rave reviews. If you are making it for children, you might want to eliminate the chili sauce.

YIELD: 24 SERVINGS

SAUCE

2 tablespoons low-fat peanut butter

½ cup fat-free plain yogurt

1 teaspoon sesame oil

4 tablespoons low-sodium soy sauce

¼ cup mirin (asian cooking wine)

⅛ teaspoon chili sauce

1 teaspoon chopped cilantro

1 tablespoon fructose

1 clove garlic, minced

1 teaspoon minced ginger

CHICKEN

6 4-ounce chicken breast halves, boned and cut into ½-inch wide strips

24 (6 inch) bamboo skewers

¼ teaspoon salt

Pepper to taste

Oil spray

Juice of 2 limes

1. Place all of the ingredients for the sauce in a blender or food processor; process until smooth and well blended. Set aside.
2. Thread the chicken strips onto skewers, starting from the short end. Once all the chicken strips are skewered, season them with salt and pepper. Place on a cookie sheet or grill and spray with oil spray and squirt lime juice over all chicken. Cook chicken for 5 minutes on each side, or until cooked through.

3. Arrange on a platter with the peanut sauce. Garnish with cilantro and lime slices.
4. Serve hot or at room temperature.

Nutrition Facts

Serving Size 2 skewers, *Calories* 53, *Fat* 1g, *Saturated Fat* 0g, *Cholesterol* 16mg, *Protein* 7g, *Carbohydrate* 3g, *Sugars* 2g, *Dietary Fiber* 0g, *Sodium* 143mg

Gayle's Feel-Good Facts

Don't feel guilty eating nuts. They are not fattening if eaten in small portions each day. Try to eat at least 4 servings (2 teaspoon of nut butter, 1 teaspoon of oil, six large or fifteen small nuts, or 1 tablespoon of seeds) daily. Shelled nuts keep for three to four months and up to a year in the freezer.

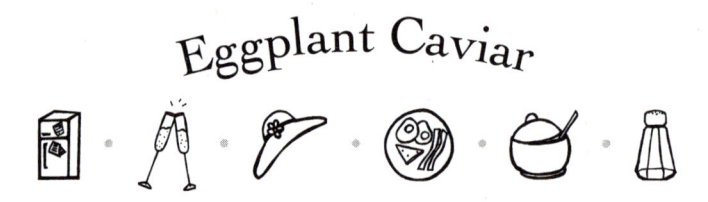

Eggplant Caviar

A perfect snack or dip to have anytime. Made of only vegetables, this dip has virtually no calories, so eat up and enjoy without any guilt! I recommend keeping it in the refrigerator to snack on anytime.

YIELD: 3 CUPS

2 medium eggplants
Sea or kosher salt
1 head garlic
1 teaspoon olive oil

2 red bell peppers
2 teaspoons fresh lemon juice
¼ cup chopped basil

2 tablespoons chopped parsley

1 teaspoon chopped thyme or ½ teaspoon dried thyme

¼ teaspoon freshly ground black pepper

Pinch of cayenne

1. Peel the eggplants and cut into ½-inch slices. Sprinkle generously with salt. Let it drain in a colander for 40 minutes. Rinse and pat dry.
2. Preheat the oven to 350 degrees. Slice off the top ¼ inch of the garlic head, to reveal the cloves. Season lightly with salt and sprinkle with 1 teaspoon of the oil. Wrap the head completely in aluminum foil.
3. Spray a baking sheet with cooking oil spray or line with parchment paper. Place the eggplant, red peppers, and garlic on the baking sheet. Roast until the eggplant is soft and golden, about 40 to 50 minutes. The garlic might need a little more time to become soft.
4. Transfer the peppers to a bowl and cover with plastic wrap. Allow the peppers to steam for 10 minutes, then remove the wrap. When the peppers are cool, peel and seed them. The skin should come off easily.
5. When the garlic is cool, squeeze the cloves into a food processor. Add the red peppers, eggplant, lemon juice, basil, parsley, and thyme. Pulse until coarsely blended. Do not puree. Season with salt, black pepper, and cayenne.

Nutrition Facts:

Serving Size 2 tablespoons, *Calories* 15, *Fat* 0g, *Saturated Fat* 0g, *Cholesterol* 0mg, *Protein* 0g, *Carbohydrate* 2g, *Sugars* 2g, *Dietary Fiber* 1g, *Sodium* 28mg

Quick Tip

When serving dip, look for whole-grain crackers or low-fat tortilla chips, if you don't make your own. You can also save yourself time by buying the premade dips and zipping them up with fresh chopped herbs. Parsley or cilantro are some herbs you can use to brighten up any store-bought dip. A squeeze of lemon juice can also help add freshness to a store-bought spread.

Classy Vegetable Spring Rolls
with Mango-Mustard Sauce

This is a satisfying treat packed with vegetables. To speed up the prep in the recipe, look for pre-shredded vegetables in the produce section of your supermarket or use a food processor for shredding and making thin slices.

YIELD: 16 LARGE SPRING ROLLS

SPRING ROLL

¼ cup honey

1 cup fresh orange juice

½ pound baked tofu, (or tofu lin), diced into small cubes (¼ inch)

32 spring roll wrappers

4 cups grated carrot

4 cups julienned nappa cabbage

1 large bell pepper, sliced thin (⅛-inch wide)

2 cups pea sprouts

4 scallions, sliced thin and long, (⅛-inch wide)

1 cup dry-roasted soy nuts

½ cup chopped cilantro

½ cup chopped basil

MANGO-MUSTARD SAUCE

2 large ripe mangos, peeled and diced (can use 2 cups frozen mango)

2 teaspoons Dijon mustard or 1 teaspoon hot Chinese mustard

¼ cup fresh orange juice

2 tablespoon cilantro

1 teaspoon low-sodium soy sauce

1. To prepare marinade for the tofu, combine the honey and orange juice in a medium bowl.
2. Chop the tofu into ¼-inch cubes and soak in the honey/orange juice mixture for at least 1 hour in the refrigerator (this can be done the night before).

3. Before preparing the spring rolls, drain the tofu from the orange juice mixture and pat dry.
4. Place each prepared filling ingredient on a separate small plate and arrange around your work surface.
5. Remove 2 spring roll wrappers from the package. Keep remaining wrappers well covered as they dry out easily. Place 1 wrapper on top of the other so that they are in the shape of a diamond. On the bottom third of the wrapper place $1/4$-cup carrot, $1/4$-cup cabbage, sprinkling of red pepper, pea sprouts, scallion, and $1/8$ of the marinated tofu. Top with 2 teaspoons of soy nuts and a pinch of the cilantro and basil.
6. Bring up the bottom part of the spring roll wrapper to cover the mixture, fold in the sides, and then continue to roll the wrapper up to form a log. Tuck in the bottom well and set aside, covered with plastic wrap, on a small nonstick or foil-lined baking sheet. Continue to assemble other rolls.
7. The rolls can keep in the refrigerator for 1 day. When ready to serve, bake at 350 degrees for 5 minutes, or until the wrapper turns golden brown and the edges are crisp. Slice in half on the diagonal to serve.
8. Prepare the sauce by mixing all the ingredients together in a blender or food processor until smooth. Place in a small dish for dipping.

Nutrition Facts:

Serving Size 1 spring roll with 2 tablespoons sauce, *Calories* 186, *Fat* 3g, *Saturated Fat* 0g, *Cholesterol* 0mg, *Protein* 10g, *Carbohydrate* 32g, *Sugars* 16g, *Dietary Fiber* 5g, *Sodium* 92mg

Tortilla Cups with Black Bean Salsa

These little tortilla cups are very cute, and can be filled with anything. The black bean salsa is popular to serve at parties, since it is a well-liked Mexican combination—black beans with tomato and seasoning.

YIELD: 48 CUPS

12 low-fat whole-wheat tortillas	½ cup diced plum tomatoes
Oil spray	1 teaspoon chopped garlic
1½ cups canned or precooked black beans	½ teaspoon cinnamon
¼ cup minced red bell pepper	2 tablespoons lime juice
¼ cup minced green bell pepper	1½ tablespoons raspberry vinegar
¼ cup minced yellow bell pepper	1 tablespoon extra virgin olive oil
½ cup minced red onion	½ teaspoon salt
2 teaspoons minced jalapeno pepper	Black pepper to taste
2 teaspoons chopped fresh cilantro	

1. Using a 3-inch round cookie cutter, cut out circles from the tortilla.
2. Place the rounds into the muffin cups of a nonstick mini-muffin pan that has been sprayed with oil.
3. Bake at 350 degrees for 5 to 10 minutes, or until firm, light brown and crisp.
4. Cool tortilla cups on a rack.
5. Combine the remaining ingredients together in a large mixing bowl. Refrigerate for 1 to 2 hours before using if possible. This helps to blend the flavors.

6. Fill the tortilla cups with 1 tablespoon of salsa, and serve cold or room temperature.

Nutrition Facts:

Serving Size 2 tortilla cups, *Calories* 74, *Fat* 2g, *Saturated Fat* 0g, *Cholesterol* 0mg, *Protein* 4g, *Carbohydrate* 10g, *Sugars* 1g, *Dietary Fiber* 5g, *Sodium* 175mg

Quick Tip

Another way to make a quick bean salsa is to simply combine a can of beans with a jar of your favorite tomato salsa. You can add the salsa to taste. Start with 1 can of beans and ½ jar of salsa. You can use the bean salsa to fill the tortilla shells as listed in the recipe on page 70. Or you can use the phyllo shells that are made by Apollo brands in the freezer case at your supermarket, or cracker type shells that are made for hor d'oeuvres, which are usually found in the specialty cracker section at gourmet stores and supermarkets.

Spicy Indonesian Shrimp Skewers

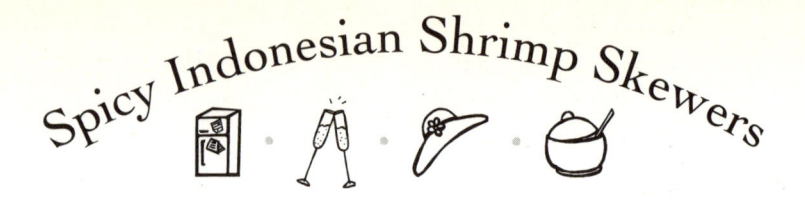

This recipe also works well with chicken, scallops, or firm tofu. To speed up your prep time, if you use shrimp, have the fish market clean and devein the shrimp and make the marinade ahead. This is a quick, tasty appetizer that is simple to prepare and can be served at room temperature, cold, or hot.

YIELD: 16 SKEWERS

- 1 cup lite coconut milk
- ½ cup chopped fresh cilantro
- 2 tablespoons fructose
- 1 tablespoon curry powder
- 1 teaspoon turmeric
- 1 jalapeno pepper, seeded and diced
- 1 tablespoon chopped garlic (about 3 cloves)
- 1 teaspoon fresh minced ginger
- 2 teaspoons fresh lime juice
- 1 teaspoon fresh chopped lemongrass (optional)
- 1 tablespoon canola oil
- 1 pound shrimp (16 large shrimp or about 22 medium shrimp), cleaned and deveined, tails intact if possible
- 16 6-inch wooden skewers or long wooden toothpicks (3 inches)
- 1 pineapple, cut into 16 1-inch cubes

1. Combine the coconut milk, cilantro, fructose, curry powder, turmeric, jalapeno, garlic, ginger, lime juice, lemongrass (optional), and oil in a blender or food processor and puree.
2. Place the cleaned shrimp in a medium bowl with the coconut-milk marinade and let soak in the refrigerator for at least 1 hour, or overnight.
3. Soak the wooden skewers in water for 30 minutes to 1 hour.
4. Skewer 1 piece of pineapple and 1 piece of shrimp per skewer.
5. Cook the skewers on the grill on medium-high heat or broil under high heat for about 4 to 6 minutes, until the shrimp is cooked.
6. Serve hot or room temperature.

Nutrition Facts:

Serving Size 1 skewer, Calories 57, Fat 2g, Saturated Fat 1g, Cholesterol 40mg, Protein 5g, Carbohydrate 5g, Sugars 4g, Dietary Fiber 0g, Sodium 51mg

4

Soups and Chili

Soups and chili are wonderful comfort foods. Great as starters, hearty soups and chili also can take center stage as a satisfying healthy lunch option. Since vegetables are so low in calories, feel free to have any vegetable soup or vegetable-based soup any time as part of a weight-management program. In spas, a technique that is used to help you stay full on less food is what I call meal layering. Meal layering is based on the premise that it takes about twenty minutes for your body to register that you are eating, so the strategy is to fill up on lower-calorie foods first, such as soup and salad, and then move on to the entrée. By the time you are digging your fork into your entrée, you are already starting to feel satiated, so you get full on fewer calories.

Look for the quick tips I have included throughout this section to shorten your prep time. Soup can take a bit of time, but when you make a soup, you are making it in such a large quantity that the perk is you get to freeze some and eat it later.

Bouquet garni (bag of garnish), in my opinion, is a must for almost every soup. You make a bouquet garni by wrapping 2 sprigs of parsley, 1 large bay leaf, and

1 pinch of thyme in a cheesecloth and tying it. It can also be wrapped up in leek leaves, but this is much harder to do.

Black Bean Soup

Black beans make a hearty, earthy soup that is great to warm you up in the cold weather. For an added kick, feel free to use hot sauce as a condiment.

YIELD: 8 CUPS

½ pound black beans, soaked overnight, or 1 16-ounce can black beans

2 medium onions

6 cloves garlic

2 cups peeled and diced carrots (about 6 carrots)

3 stalks celery, sliced (1 cup)

2 teaspoons olive oil

1 tablespoon ground cumin

1 teaspoon ground paprika

¼ cup chopped fresh cilantro

6 cups vegetable broth

½ cup chopped fresh tomato

2 bay leaves

1 tablespoon cider vinegar

1 teaspoon kosher salt

2 teaspoons black pepper

½ cup low-fat or fat-free sour cream (optional) for garnish

1. To soak the beans, place them in a large pot and cover with water. Make sure there is two times the amount of water to the number of beans. It doesn't matter how much water you use as long as it covers the beans well. The more water the better. Let sit overnight. Alternatively, you can use canned drained beans.
2. In a large soup pot, sauté the onion, garlic, carrot, and celery in the olive oil. Add the cumin, paprika, and cilantro and stir for 30 seconds. Add the beans,

vegetable broth, tomato, and bay leaves. Cook until the beans are tender if using fresh beans, approximately 30 minutes. Add the vinegar and cook 10 minutes more.
3. Purée in batches and add the salt and pepper to taste.
4. Serve with a sprinkle of the chopped cilantro. As an option you can put on top of each serving a tablespoon of low-fat sour cream and sprinkle the cilantro on top of the sour cream for taste and color.

Nutrition Facts:

Serving Size 1 cup, *Calories* 151, *Fat* 2g, *Saturated Fat* 0g, *Cholesterol* 1mg, *Protein* 9g, *Carbohydrate* 26g, *Sugars* 6g, *Dietary Fiber* 7g, *Sodium* 914mg

Carrot-Orange Soup with Ginger

This sweet soup is good any time of the year. It can be served hot or room temperature.

YIELD: 6 CUPS

3 small onions, diced
1 teaspoon canola oil
6 cups diced carrots
2 tablespoons minced ginger
6 cups vegetable broth

1 cup orange juice (preferably fresh)
1 teaspoon sugar
¼ teaspoon salt
½ teaspoon white pepper
¼ cup chopped cilantro

1. In a large soup pot, sauté the onion in oil until soft and translucent. Once the onions are soft, add the carrots and ginger and sauté for 1 minute.
2. Add the vegetable broth and cook until the carrots are tender.
3. Purée in a food processor or blender, return to the soup pot, and add the orange juice and sugar.
4. Season with salt and pepper.
5. If soup is too thick add more broth or water to thin it out.
6. Sprinkle soup with fresh cilantro before serving.

Nutrition Facts:

Serving Size 1 cup, *Calories* 132, *Fat* 2g, *Saturated Fat* 0g, *Cholesterol* 0mg, *Protein* 5g, *Carbohydrate* 27g, *Sugars* 20g, *Dietary Fiber* 5g, *Sodium* 978mg

Quick Tip for Soups

Also, for bean soups, canned beans really help to speed up the cooking process. The salt in a can of beans is mostly in the liquid, so simply rinse off the beans in a strainer before using.

Gayle's Feel-Good Facts

The orange color of carrots is an indication of their high content of carotenes, in particular betacarotene. People who eat foods rich in carotenes have a lower risk of heart disease, stroke, cataracts, and some forms of cancer. Betacarotene is not destroyed by heat. Betacarotene is also high in other orange vegetables, including pumpkin, winter squash, and sweet potatoes.

Creamy Broccoli Soup with Cheddar

Typically, creamy soups are off-limits if you are looking to reduce fat in your diet and watch your cholesterol. However, the potato in this soup helps to thicken it right up and doesn't contribute any fat. Plus, broccoli is one of the most popular anticancer vegetables.

YIELD: 10 CUPS

2 pounds broccoli

1 small onion, coarsely chopped

1 leek, chopped, white only

1 carrot, chopped

1 stalk celery, chopped

1 teaspoon canola oil

4 cups vegetable broth

Bouquet garni (cheesecloth filled with a bay leaf, a pinch of dried thyme, and 2 sprigs of parsley, tied with twine)

3 cups water

1 large Idaho potato, peeled and diced

½ teaspoon salt, optional

½ teaspoon black pepper

1 cup evaporated skim milk

2 cups grated low-fat soy cheddar cheese or low-fat cheddar cheese

1. Trim the broccoli, peel and chop the stems, and chop the heads into small florets.
2. Sauté the onions, leeks, carrots, and celery in oil for 5 minutes to sweat.
3. Add the broth, bouquet garni, water, and potato. Bring to a boil and lower the heat to a simmer. Add the broccoli. Cook until the broccoli is tender, about 20 to 25 minutes.
4. Remove from the heat, remove the bouquet garni, and purée the soup in a blender or food processor.

5. Return the soup to the pot, and add the evaporated skim milk and cheddar cheese. Stir until cheese melts.
6. Season with salt and pepper. Serve hot.

Nutrition Facts:

Serving Size 1 cup, Calories 122, Fat 3g, Saturated Fat 1g, Cholesterol 6mg, Protein 12g, Carbohydrate 15g, Sugars 8g, Dietary Fiber 4g, Sodium 715mg.

Quick Tip

Use frozen cut vegetables for soups instead of fresh if you want to reduce your prep time.

Decadent Corn Chowder

An easy soup to prepare, especially when you use the frozen corn, this soup is a sweet addition to any meal.

YIELD: 16 CUPS

4 ears of fresh corn on the cob (or use 3 cups of frozen sweet corn)

1 cup chopped onions

1 leek, chopped

2 sprigs fresh thyme

¼ cup white wine

½ cup chopped celery

1 cup chopped carrots

3 cups vegetable broth

1 cup red potatoes, chopped into ½-inch pieces (about 2 to 3 potatoes)

2 sprigs fresh parsley

1 can (12 ounces) evaporated skim milk

½ teaspoon Tabasco (optional)

½ teaspoon Worcestershire

¼ teaspoon salt

¼ teaspoon white pepper

1. With a knife, remove the fresh corn from the cob by slicing down the cob from top to bottom. Save the cobs and set the corn aside. Or use 3 cups thawed frozen corn.
2. In a large soup pot, sweat the onions, leeks, and thyme in white wine until soft. Add the celery and carrots. Sweat 2 minutes.
3. Add the vegetable broth and all of the corncobs. Bring to boil and let simmer for 10 minutes.
4. Add potatoes and cook until almost soft, about 8 minutes.
5. Remove the thyme and corncobs.
6. Add the corn kernels and simmer until the potatoes are tender but not mushy, about 15 minutes.
7. Purée the soup mixture in a blender and return to the pot.
8. Add the evaporated milk and extra broth or water if the soup is too thick.
9. Season with Tabasco, Worcestershire, salt, and pepper.
10. Serve hot or cold.

Optional toppings for corn chowder:
- Crab Meat—2 tablespoons per person or 1 cup total for recipe.
- Jalepeno—Slice a fresh jalapeno and put 2 to 3 slices on top of the chowder before serving (for recipe use 4 jalepenos). Do not serve seeds as they can leave your mouth burning.

Nutrition Facts:

Serving Size 1 cup, *Calories* 114, *Fat* 0g, *Saturated Fat* 0g, *Cholesterol* 1mg, *Protein* 6g, *Carbohydrate* 23g, *Sugars* 7g, *Dietary Fiber* 3g, *Sodium* 475mg

Gazpacho Soup

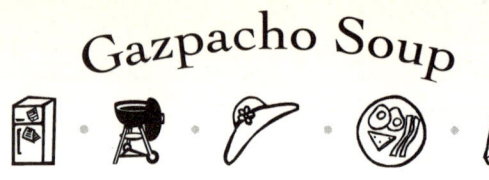

This is an excellent recipe for a favorite cold summer soup. I really love having this for lunch on a hot summer day. Feel free to serve it hot in the cooler months. It is chockful of healthy vegetables, plus the tomatoes provide you with plenty of lycopene, an antioxidant that helps prevent prostate cancer and heart disease.

YIELD: 12 CUPS

3 slices soft wheat bread, crusts removed

4 cloves garlic

Juice of 2 lemons (about 2 tablespoons)

Juice of 1 lime (about 1 tablespoon)

1 28-ounce can peeled whole tomatoes, seeded

2 28-ounce cans peeled whole tomatoes without seeds and juice

2 bunches scallions, white parts only

3 seedless cucumbers, peeled and cut into $\frac{1}{4}$-inch dice

1 green bell peppers, seeded and diced

1 red bell pepper, seeded and diced

1 yellow bell pepper, seeded and diced

1 large can or bottle (46 ounces) of V-8 juice

2½ tablespoons sherry wine vinegar

2 teaspoons extra virgin olive oil

Dash of Tabasco sauce

½ teaspoon salt

½ teaspoon black pepper

½ teaspoon sugar, optional

1. Place the bread, garlic, and lemon and lime juices in a blender or food processor and process to a smooth paste.
2. In a large bowl, add all the vegetables to the bread paste and toss to combine. Stir in the V-8, then the vinegar, oil, Tabasco, salt, and pepper. If the soup tastes too tart, feel free to add the sugar.
3. Purée half the soup in the food processor or blender and combine with the un-puréed ingredients. Refrigerate until very cold.
4. Serve cold.

Nutrition Facts:

Serving Size 1 cup, *Calories* 73, *Fat* 0g, *Saturated Fat* 0g, *Cholesterol* 0mg, *Protein* 2g, *Carbohydrate* 15g, *Sugars* 8g, *Dietary Fiber* 4g, *Sodium* 64mg

Quick Tip

If you are really short on time and want to serve soup, you can buy premade canned soups and "doctor them up" with fresh herbs and seasoning in order to make them taste more homemade. Good herbs to use for this purpose include chopped fresh parsley, chervil, tarragon, dill, and if it is a hearty bean soup, thyme works well. Other seasonings to try are fresh chopped garlic or garlic powder, onion powder, dried bouquet garni, salt, pepper, and hot sauce (Tabasco). If you are having trouble knowing what herb to pick, refer to the herb charts on pages 21–22.

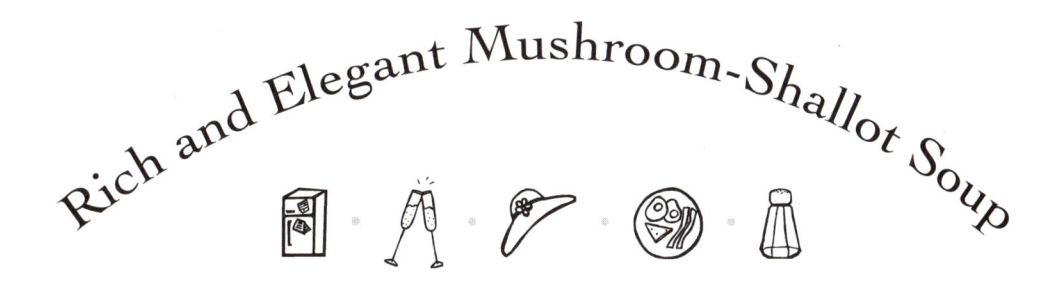

Rich and Elegant Mushroom-Shallot Soup

This is a delicious, hearty soup that is very low in calories. To save time on this recipe, purchase already chopped mushrooms in the produce section of your supermarket.

YIELD: 8 CUPS

2 shallots, finely chopped

1 leek, white only, finely chopped

1 tablespoon olive oil

¼ cup dry white wine

2 portabella mushrooms, chopped
1 pound Oregon cepes, chopped
¼ pound porcini, chopped
½ pound shitake, chopped
3 cups vegetable broth

3 sprigs tarragon, chopped
2 sprigs thyme, chopped
½ teaspoon salt
Black pepper to taste.

1. In a large soup pot over medium heat saute the shallots and leeks in olive oil until translucent or slightly browned, about 2 to 3 minutes. Add the white wine and allow to cook for 2 minutes.
2. Add the chopped mushrooms and vegetable broth and raise the heat to medium-high.
3. Bring the soup to a simmer and let it cook for 20 to 30 minutes.
4. Purée in a blender or food processor with a steel blade until well mixed and smooth. Pour the puréed soup back in the pot. Stir in the herbs, salt, and pepper. If soup is too thick, add additional broth or water to achieve desired consistency.
5. Bring to a boil. Serve hot.

Nutrition Facts:

Serving Size 1 cup, Calories 115, Fat 3g, Saturated Fat 0g, Cholesterol 0mg, Protein 9g, Carbohydrate 14g, Sugars 2g, Dietary Fiber 5g, Sodium 554mg

Gayle's Feel-Good Facts

Mushrooms, while grouped in the vegetable family, are really considered a fungus, and a healthy one at that. Research has shown that cooked mushrooms contain antibacterial and antitumor substances, particularly those used in Asian cooking such as shitake, enoki, and oyster. Since they grow close to the soil, mushrooms are rich in minerals such as iron, zinc, and copper.

Hearty Vegetable Soup

Have this soup anytime as a starter, snack, or part of a meal. Since vegetables are so low in calories and high in protective plant nutrients, they provide an excellent way to fill up on a high-quality food.

YIELD: 8 CUPS

1 14-ounce can plum tomatoes in their juice

2 teaspoons olive oil

1 small onion, diced

4 medium leeks, white part only, cleaned and sliced into rounds

2 stalks celery, diced

1 clove garlic, minced

6 cups vegetable broth, or enough to cover vegetables

1 small head green cabbage, shredded

4 carrots, peeled and diced

4 medium red potatoes, skins on, diced

2 turnips, diced

1 tablespoon chopped fresh parsley

½ teaspoon dried thyme

¼ teaspoon dried oregano

1 bay leaf

½ pound green beans, cut into 1-inch pieces

Freshly ground black pepper

Pinch of sugar or fructose

1. Coarsely chop the plum tomatoes and set aside. Save the juice of the tomatoes.
2. Heat a large soup pot over medium heat, add the oil followed by the onion, leeks, celery, and garlic.
3. Cover and cook over medium heat until the vegetables are wilted, adding some broth if necessary to prevent burning.
4. Add the cabbage and cook for 5 minutes, or until it begins to soften. Add the tomatoes and their juice, the remaining broth, carrots, potatoes, turnips, and herbs.
5. Cover and cook until the carrots and potatoes are barely soft. Skim the foam

from the surface of the soup occasionally. Add the green beans and cook until just tender. Adjust the seasonings and serve.

Nutrition Facts:

Serving Size 1 cup, *Calories* 107, *Fat* 1g, *Saturated Fat* 0g, *Cholesterol* 0mg, *Protein* 3g, *Carbohydrate* 22g, *Sugars* 0g, *Dietary Fiber* 2g, *Sodium* 132mg

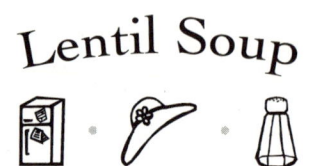

Lentil Soup

Of all the beans, lentils are some of the more popular because of their mild flavor and easy digestibility, plus they cook quickly, so they are easier to use. Enjoy this hearty soup for lunch or a starter for dinner.

YIELD: 8 CUPS

1 cup chopped onions	4 cups vegetable broth
1 clove minced garlic	Bouquet garni
1 cup chopped carrot	½ cup canned chopped tomatoes in juice
1 leek (white part only), chopped	1 tablespoon olive oil
¼ cup chopped celery	½ teaspoon salt
1 lb. dried lentils (feel free to choose green, yellow, or red)	½ teaspoon pepper
	¼ cup chopped parsley (optional)

1. In a large soup pot, sauté the onion, garlic, carrots, leek, and celery in olive oil to sweat, about 8 minutes.
2. Add the lentils, vegetable broth, bouquet garni, and tomatoes to the pot and bring to a boil. Cover, reduce heat, and simmer for 45 minutes.
3. Season with salt and pepper before servings.
4. Top each bowl of soup with a sprinkle of fresh parsley.

Nutrition Facts:

Serving Size 1 *cup, Calories* 220, *Fat* 3g, *Saturated Fat* 0g, *Cholesterol* 0mg, *Protein* 16g, *Carbohydrate* 37g, *Sugars* 9g, *Dietary Fiber* 16g, *Sodium* 1161mg

Gayle's Feel-Good Facts

Dried beans (legumes) are high in protein and fiber. For diabetics and those who crave carbs, the soluble fiber found in beans helps to regulate blood sugar, keeping levels more even. The high-protein content of beans also helps keep you satiated longer.

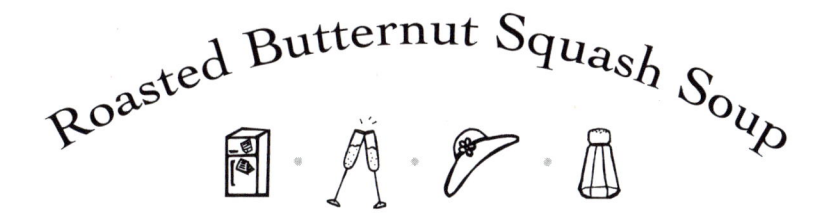

Roasted Butternut Squash Soup

A sweet, warm flavor, butternut squash makes an excellent soup for the fall and winter. This soup should also help you boost your immune system, as one cup contains 50 percent of your vitamin A requirement and ample vitamin C.

YIELD: 10 CUPS

2 medium-large butternut squash (about 4 cups) (can substitute 1 to 2 cups of squash for pumpkin purée if desired, then use only 1 squash)

2 carrots, chopped

½ medium onion, chopped

1 leek, chopped, whites only

1 stalk of celery, chopped

1 tablespoon olive oil

4 teaspoons curry powder

6 cups of vegetable broth

Bouquet garni

½ teaspoon chopped thyme or ¼ teaspoon ground dried thyme

1 tablespoon dry sherry

¾ cup applesauce, all natural, unsweetened

¼ cup evaporated skim milk (optional)

Juice of ½ orange

¼ teaspoon salt

Black pepper, ground

1. Preheat the oven to 400 degrees.
2. Slice the squash in half and place facedown on a cookie sheet that is either non-stick or has foil or parchment lining the pan.
3. Cook for 1 hour.
4. Allow the squash to cool. Remove the seeds and scoop out the contents of the squash for use in the soup.
5. In a large soup pot sauté the carrots, onions, leeks, and celery in 1 tablespoon of olive oil for about 5 minutes. Add the curry and stir for 30 seconds.
6. Add the squash purée and broth. Mix well, so that the purée is well blended in the vegetable broth. Add the bouquet garni and thyme.
7. Bring to a boil, then reduce to a simmer. Cook for 20 minutes. Remove the bouquet garni, place the soup in a food processor or blender, and blend the soup until it is smooth. If the soup is too thick, add more broth to reach the desired consistency. Return the puréed soup to the pot, add the sherry, applesauce, and evaporated skim milk. Bring to a boil, reduce to a simmer, add the orange juice, salt, and pepper. Serve hot.

Nutrition Facts:

Serving Size 1 cup, *Calories* 97, *Fat* 2g, *Saturated Fat* 0g, *Cholesterol* 0mg, *Protein* 3g, *Carbohydrate* 19g, *Sugars* 9g, *Dietary Fiber* 4g, *Sodium* 682mg

Mediterranean Roasted Red Pepper Soup

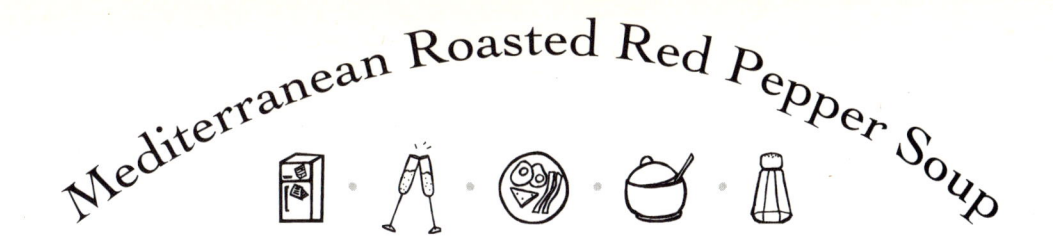

The roasted peppers add an excellent sweet woodsy flavor to this lite soup. Since this soup is primarily vegetable based, the calories are minimal, so enjoy this soup any time, and don't hesitate to have it as a snack.

YIELD: 6 CUPS

1 small onion, diced

1 small leek, finely chopped

1 tablespoon olive oil

1 celery stalk, diced

3 carrots, diced

4 cups vegetable broth

Bouquet garni

4 large red peppers, roasted and peeled

1 can (6 ounces) tomato purée

Salt to taste

Black pepper to taste

8-ounce container plain nonfat yogurt

¼ cup chopped basil

1. In a large soup pot, sweat the onion and leak in oil until translucent over a medium flame. Add the celery and carrots and cook an additional 1 to 2 minutes.
2. Add the vegetable broth and bouquet garni. Cook for 15 minutes, until the carrots are soft.
3. Add the roasted peppers and tomato purée and simmer for 10 minutes.
4. Remove from the heat and remove the bouquet garni. Purée the soup in a blender or food processor.
5. To reheat, place back in the pot and bring to a boil. Season with salt and pepper.
6. To serve, place a rounded tablespoon of plain yogurt in the middle and sprinkle with chopped basil.

Nutrition Facts:

Serving Size 1 cup, Calories 145, Fat 3g, Saturated Fat 0g, Cholesterol 0mg, Protein 6g, Carbohydrate 27g, Sugars 18g, Dietary Fiber 5g, Sodium 120mg

Gayle's Feel-Good Facts

Red peppers are sweet and bursting with the antioxidants vitamin A and vitamin C. When they are roasted they take on a smoked flavor that adds a nice smokey sweet taste to any recipe.

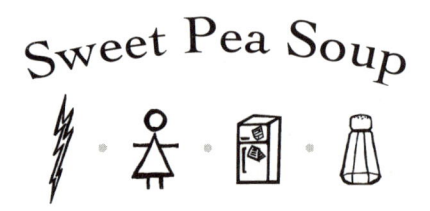

Sweet Pea Soup

Puréed peas make a lovely rich-tasting soup that is easy to prepare and good to eat any time of the year. As a legume, like beans, peas are rich in protein.

YIELD: 6 CUPS

½ small sweet white onion, sliced

1 large leek (white part only), chopped

1 tablespoon canola oil

12 ounces peas, frozen and thawed

2 cups vegetable broth

6 ounces plain yogurt (nonfat)

1 teaspoon sugar

Dash of Tabasco

¼ cup mint leaves, chopped

Pinch of salt

Black pepper to taste

1. In a large soup pot, sauté the onion and leeks in canola oil until soft.
2. Add the peas and broth and bring to a boil. When it reaches a boil, turn down to a simmer and add the yogurt and sugar.
3. Cook until the peas are soft.
4. Before serving, season with Tabasco, mint, salt, and pepper. Serve hot.

Nutrition Facts:

Serving Size 1 cup, *Calories* 115, *Fat* 3g, *Saturated Fat* 0g, *Cholesterol* 0mg, *Protein* 6g, *Carbohydrate* 18g, *Sugars* 11g, *Dietary Fiber* 4g, *Sodium* 470mg

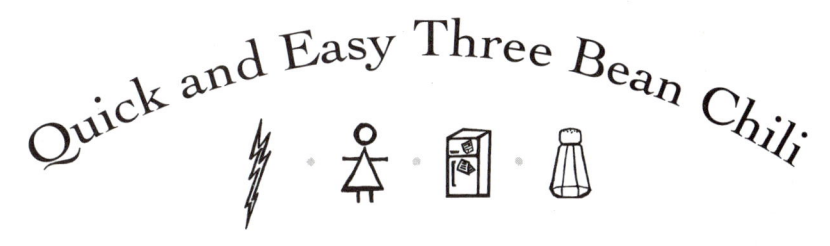

Quick and Easy Three Bean Chili

This chili is simple to make and scrumptious to eat. Although it is vegetarian, the bulgur gives it a meaty texture, so much so that many people think there is meat in it.

YIELD: 12 CUPS

1 teaspoon canola oil

2 green bell peppers, cubed

2 medium onions, cubed

2 teaspoons dried basil

2 teaspoons dried cumin

1½ teaspoons chili powder

1 teaspoon oregano

¼ teaspoon cayenne or jalapeno powder

1 28-ounce can Italian plum tomatoes, chopped

2 cups water

1 teaspoon salt

1 teaspoon sugar

1 cup bulgur wheat

1 15-ounce can black beans, drained

1 15-ounce can pinto beans, drained

1 15-ounce can red beans, drained

1 cup frozen corn kernels

¼ cup chopped cilantro

1. Add the oil to a broth pot or Dutch oven and sear the peppers and onions over high heat. Cook 2 minutes then stir in the basil, cumin, chili powder, oregano, and cayenne and cook 30 seconds. Add the tomatoes, water, salt, and sugar.
2. Add the bulgur, stir well, lower the heat, and simmer, covered, until the bulgur is cooked, about 20 minutes. Stir in the beans, corn, and cilantro.
3. Cook 10 more minutes.

Nutrition Facts:

Serving Size 1 cup, *Calories* 225, *Fat* 1.5g, *Saturated Fat* 0g, *Cholesterol* 0mg, *Protein* 23g, *Carbohydrate* 45g, *Sugars* 7g, *Dietary Fiber* 12g, *Sodium* 323mg

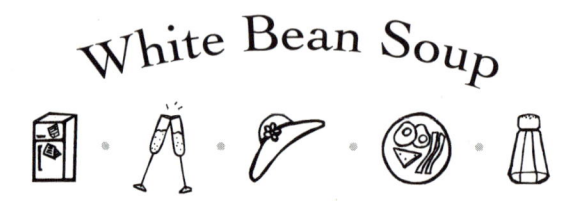

White Bean Soup

The robust herbs thyme and sage impart a wonderful flare to this traditional bean soup.

YIELD: 8 CUPS

1 teaspoon oil

1 small leek, diced

1 small onion, diced

2 stalks celery, diced

3 medium carrots, diced

3 cloves garlic, minced

¼ cup white wine

8 cups chicken or vegetable broth

1 bay leaf

1 teaspoon finely chopped thyme

1 teaspoon finely chopped sage

1 pound cannellini beans, canned

¼ cup finely chopped basil

Salt, to taste

1 teaspoon black pepper

1. Heat the oil in a large pot. Add the leek, onion, celery, carrots, and garlic.
2. Cook, stirring, for about 1 minute, then add the wine. Cook until the onions are soft and golden.
3. Add the broth, bay leaf, thyme, and sage.
4. Add the beans and bring to a boil. Lower the heat to medium and simmer until the beans are just tender, about 1 to 2 hours.
5. Remove the bay leaf and transfer half of the mixture, in batches, to a blender and purée.
6. Return to the pot. Add the fresh basil and stir well. Season with salt and pepper.

Nutrition Facts:

Serving Size 1 cup, *Calories* 204, *Fat* .5g, *Saturated Fat* 0g, *Cholesterol* 0mg, *Protein* 12g, *Carbohydrate* 31g, *Sugars* 4g, *Dietary Fiber* 4g, *Sodium* 282mg

5

Salads

Salads make excellent meals or starters and can be extremely satisfying. I have compiled a group of salads that I think are a nice balance of vegetables, proteins, and grains. When focusing on health, often it is the dressing on the salad that adds all the extra and unnecessary calories from fat. I have listed a number of traditional salads lightened up, so you can have your favorites without guilt. I have also included easy low-fat dressings you can make and keep in the refrigerator. A serving of dressing is two tablespoons. Feel free to use more if you like, but be aware that the calories can add up. By putting the right flavor combinations together, a salad can offer a very pleasing dining experience that both looks colorful and is bursting with freshness and flavor!

Low-Fat Caesar Salad

This salad can be a crisp, delicious starter. Topped with grilled shrimp or roasted chicken breast, it makes a more substantial entrée salad. A regular Caesar salad is usually packed with calories and fat from the dressing and can have as many as 600 calories and 11 grams of fat. With only 58 calories and 1 gram of fat, this recipe gives you a huge savings.

YIELD: 4 SERVINGS

1 large head of romaine lettuce, torn into bite-size pieces

1 cup of Low-Fat Caesar Salad Dressing (recipe page 117)

2 tablespoons grated Parmesan cheese

1 cup whole-grain croutons

Freshly ground black pepper to taste

1. In a large bowl combine the lettuce, salad dressing, Parmesan cheese, and croutons.
2. Season with black pepper to taste.

Nutrition Facts:

Serving Size 1/4 salad, Calories 46, Fat 2g, Saturated Fat 0g, Cholesterol 4mg, Protein 4g, Carbohydrate 4g, Sugars 2g, Dietary Fiber 1g, Sodium 182mg

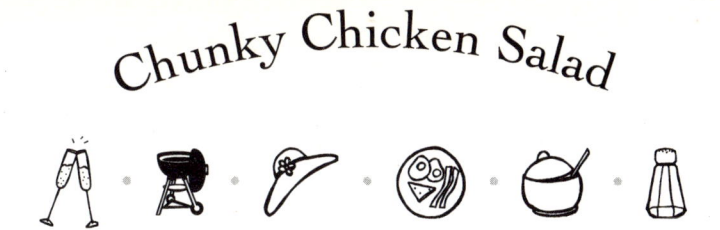

Chunky Chicken Salad
with Celery, Apples, and Walnuts

The fresh variety of tastes created by the celery, apples, and the Lemon-Tarragon Buttermilk Dressing make this a very refreshing and filling entrée salad.

YIELD: 6 SERVINGS

SALAD

2 cups chicken broth, fat-free or defatted

6 3-ounce boneless chicken breasts

½ cup finely chopped walnuts

1½ heads Boston or butterhead lettuce

2 celery stalks, sliced

1 Granny Smith apple, cored and cubed

DRESSING

1 cup Lemon-Tarragon Buttermilk Dressing (recipe page 112)

½ teaspoon dry mustard

¼ cup fat-free mayonnaise

1. In a large saucepan, bring the chicken broth to a simmer, add the chicken breasts, and poach until the chicken is cooked, about 12 to 14 minutes.
2. Transfer the cooked chicken to a cutting board to cool.
3. Toast the walnuts by broiling them in a toaster or regular oven for 3 to 5 minutes. Be careful not to keep them too close to a flame or they may catch fire. Once cooled, chop.
4. Wash and tear the lettuce into bite-size pieces. Set aside.
5. Cut the chicken breast into bite-size pieces and place in a large mixing bowl with the celery, apples, and walnuts. Mix until well combined.

6. Combine dressing ingredients in a medium bowl and mix well. Toss dressing in with chicken mixture.
7. On each plate place a cup of lettuce and then the chicken in the center.

Nutrition Facts:

Serving Size 1/6 of salad, Calories 235, Fat 8g, Saturated Fat 1g, Cholesterol 50mg, Protein 21g, Carbohydrate 13g, Sugars 9g, Dietary Fiber 2g, Sodium 201mg

Gayle's Feel-Good Facts

Walnuts are high in protective omega-3 fats. Sprinkling them and other nuts in the foods you eat will help you insure that you are taking in these essential fats daily. Nuts are healthy: It is eating too many that can pack on the pounds, so use them and seeds more as a condiment than a main snack.

Crab and Avocado Salad

This is a lovely, light, and tasty salad that is packed with vitamin C from the citrus and red pepper and good healthy plant fats from the avocado oil.

YIELD: 4 SERVINGS

DRESSING

2 tablespoons fresh lime juice

2 tablespoons fresh lemon juice

1 teaspoon chopped fresh cilantro

4 tablespoons pineapple juice

Dash of Tabasco

½ teaspoon Old Bay Seasoning

1 tablespoon canola oil

SALAD

¼ cup sweet red pepper, diced

½ avocado, peeled and diced

1 medium tomato (about 1/2 cup), diced

12 ounces fresh lump crabmeat (choose from Dungeness, King, or blue), picked over for shell pieces

½ head of dark green lettuce, shredded

1. Combine the dressing ingredients and set aside.
2. Mix the pepper, avocado, and tomato in a medium mixing bowl until well combined. Fold in the crabmeat, mixing gently.
3. Place a cup of shredded lettuce in a large mixing bowl and toss with ¼ cup of the salad dressing.
4. Divide the crabmeat into 4 servings and place on top of the lettuce.
5. Pour 1 tablespoon of the dressing on top of the crabmeat on each plate and serve extra dressing on the side.

Nutrition Facts:

Serving Size ¼ *salad, Calories* 180, *Fat* 8.5g, *Saturated Fat* 1g, *Cholesterol* 76mg, *Protein* 19g, *Carbohydrate* 8g, *Sugars* 4g, *Dietary Fiber* 2g, *Sodium* 290mg

Quick Tip for Salads

Like soups, you can purchase precut vegetables to speed up your prep time for salads. Also, feel free to purchase low-fat or fat-free dressings and sauces that are similar to what is used in the recipe, if you are short on time. The recipe will taste a bit different, but it probably will still taste good. You can distinguish a low-fat dressing or marinade by reading the Nutrition Facts label. If it is low-fat, it will have 3 grams of total fat or less.

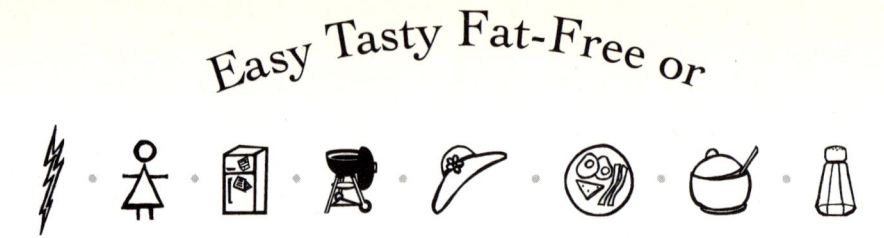

Easy Tasty Fat-Free or Low-Fat Coleslaw — Your Choice

Great for barbeques! To make this recipe even easier you can use the prepared coleslaw (a bag of shredded cabbage and carrots) sold in the produce section of the supermarket. It will keep for three days covered in the refrigerator. I like to use this as a snack because it is so low in calories.

YIELD: 5 SERVINGS

DRESSING

½ cup fat-free or low-fat mayonnaise

2 tablespoons apple cider vinegar

2½ tablespoons honey or fructose

1 teaspoon Dijon mustard (optional)

½ teaspoon salt

Pinch of ground white pepper

1 teaspoon celery seed

SLAW

¼ medium green cabbage, shredded

½ small red cabbage, shredded

3 carrots, peeled and grated

1 small jicama, peeled and grated (optional)

1. Combine all dressing ingredients in a bowl and stir together.
2. Add the vegetables to the dressing and toss well.
3. Refrigerate until ready to serve.

Nutrition Facts for the low-fat version:

Serving Size 1 cup, Calories 140, Fat 2g, Saturated Fat 0g, Cholesterol 0mg, Protein 3g, Carbohydrate 32g, Sugars 21g, Dietary Fiber 7g, Sodium 524mg

> ### Gayle's Feel-Good Facts
>
> You can't go wrong filling up on this coleslaw to help you curb your appetite if you are trying to lose weight. Cabbage is a member of the cruciferous family and like its other family members—broccoli, brussels sprouts, cauliflower—contains indols, plant compounds that fight cancer.

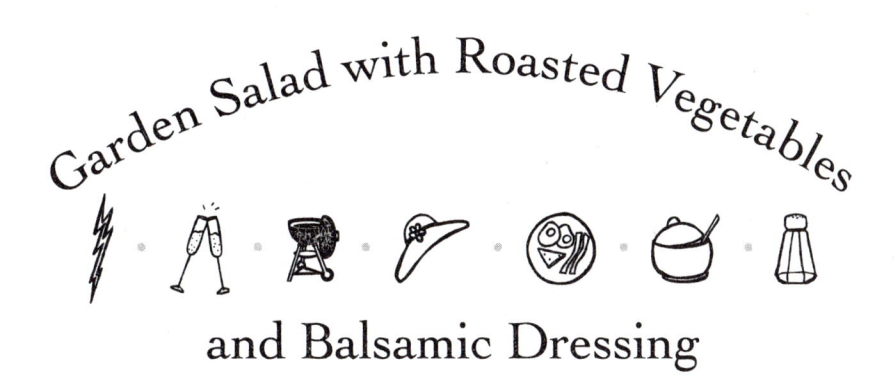

Garden Salad with Roasted Vegetables and Balsamic Dressing

The roasted vegetables jazz up this green salad with their sweet warm flavors.

YIELD: 6 SERVINGS

1 box grape tomatoes

1 medium red onion, sliced thin

2 large red peppers, sliced in quarters

1 pound baby mixed greens

1 cup shredded basil leaves

1 cup Low-Fat Balsamic Vinaigrette (page 113)

1. Line two small baking sheets with foil. Place the grape tomatoes on one baking sheet and the red onion and pepper on the other. Roast in the oven at

400 degrees, approximately 10 minutes for the tomatoes and 8 minutes for the onion and pepper. The vegetables will be soft and slightly browned when done.

2. While the vegetables are in the oven, clean and dry the greens. Mix the lettuce in a large salad bowl with the shredded basil leaves.
3. When the vegetables are roasted, take them out of the oven and cool. Slice the red pepper into thin slices. Mix the roasted vegetables with the lettuce leaves.
4. Toss with balsamic salad dressing and serve.

Nutrition Facts:

Serving Size 1/4 *salad, Calories* 119, *Fat* 3g, *Saturated Fat* 0g, *Cholesterol* 0mg, *Protein* 9g, *Carbohydrate* 18g, *Sugars* 4g, *Dietary Fiber* 5g, *Sodium* 127mg

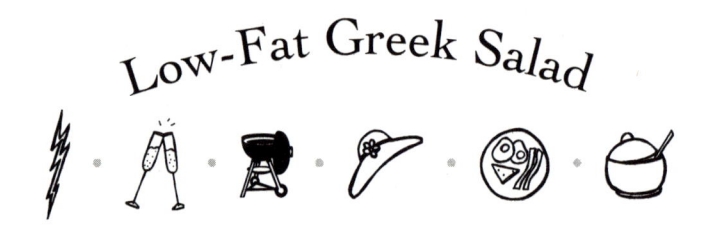

Low-Fat Greek Salad

A light version of this favorite Greek starter or entrée salad, you save calories by using low-fat cheese and fat-free dressing.

YIELD: 6 SERVINGS

1 head romaine lettuce

3/4 cup Fresh Herb Vinaigrette (page 116)

Juice of 1/2 lemon

1 teaspoon oregano, dried

1 cucumber, peeled and halved

1/4 medium red onion, thinly sliced

15 grape tomatoes, halved

Six Kalamata olives, pitted and sliced

4 ounces low-fat feta cheese, crumbled

Black pepper to taste

1. Wash and trim the lettuce of all dark spots. Dry and tear lettuce leaves into bite-size pieces. Set aside in a large salad bowl.
2. In a small bowl combine the Fresh Herb Vinaigrette with the juice of ½ lemon and the oregano.
3. Combine the cucumbers, red onions, tomatoes, and olives with the lettuce and toss well to combine.
4. Add the dressing to the salad bowl and toss well to combine.
5. Sprinkle the feta over the top. When serving, first toss the feta into the salad to combine. If making separate salad plates, plate out the salad and then sprinkle the feta and black pepper on top of each salad.

Nutrition Facts:

Serving Size ⅙ *salad, Calories* 88, *Fat* 3g, *Saturated Fat* 1g, *Cholesterol* 6mg, *Protein* 6g, *Carbohydrate* 9g, *Sugars* 1g, *Dietary Fiber* 2g, *Sodium* 608mg

Gayle's Feel-Good Facts

When seeking out low-fat cheeses, look for them in the cheese specialty case at your market. Some brands to look for include Cabot, Alpine Lace, Kraft, and Coach Farm. Many cheeses are lite or reduced, and not low-fat, so they will have a bit more than 3 grams of fat per serving. Check the recipe and look for the lowest-fat cheese you can find. But I would avoid cooking with fat-free hard cheese unless you are very restricted in your diet due to a medical condition, because fat-free cheese doesn't melt as well.

Mixed Bean Salad

A hearty salad and side. This mixed bean salad is a great source of fiber and protein.

YIELD: 12 SERVINGS

1 pound fresh green beans, trimmed and cleaned

1 can cooked red beans or 15 ounces freshly cooked

1 can cannellini beans or 15 ounces freshly cooked

12 diced ripe cherry tomatoes

1 cup chopped scallion

1 can black-eyed peas or 15 ounces freshly cooked

1 cup Low-Fat Balsamic Vinaigrette (page 113)

¼ cup julienned basil leaves

¼ cup chopped flat-leaf parsley

1. Cook the green beans in a large pot of salted boiling water until al dente, about 3 minutes. Drain the beans and refresh in a large bowl of ice water. Let stand until cool, then drain and pat dry. Cut the beans into 2-inch pieces.
2. Drain the red beans, cannellini, and black-eyed peas in a sieve or colander and rinse with cold water. Then pat dry with a paper towel to pick up excess moisture.
3. Combine the fresh and canned (or cooked) beans in a large bowl, add the tomatoes and scallions, and toss to combine. Add the Low-Fat Balsamic Vinaigrette and toss again to mix the dressing well.
4. Garnish with basil and parsley.

Nutrition Facts:

Serving Size 1 cup, Calories 138, Fat 0g, Saturated Fat 0g, Cholesterol 0mg, Protein 11g, Carbohydrate 40g, Sugars 8g, Dietary Fiber 13g, Sodium 310mg

> **Gayle's Feel-Good Facts**
>
> Parsley is known to aid digestion, plus it is high in folate and vitamin C. Use it liberally in salads, not just as a garnish.

Mixed Green Salad with Pear and Goat Cheese

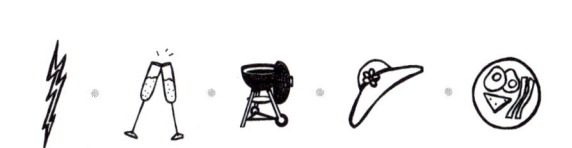

I like this recipe because of how the fruity taste of the pear complements the tangy, salty taste of the goat cheese. This is a great starter.

YIELD: 4 SERVINGS

SALAD

- 4 cups mixed greens (baby mixed greens or you can mix your own—green leaf lettuce, baby spinach, and romaine are a good combination)
- 4 ounces low-fat goat cheese crumble
- 1 Bosc pear, thinly sliced
- ½ cup pine nuts, toasted

DRESSING

- ½ cup Low-Fat Caesar Salad Dressing (page 117)
- ½ cup of Low-Fat Balsamic Vinaigrette (page 113)

1. In a large salad bowl, mix together all the salad ingredients except the pine nuts.
2. Mix the two salad dressings together. If you want to use store bought dressing,

you can purchase a low-fat Caesar and low-fat Italian dressing and combine the two. Toss with the salad and top with the pine nuts.

3. If you are plating the salad, toss the salad dressing with the greens, sprinkle the cheese and pear slices on each salad, and sprinkle pine nuts on each before serving.

Nutrition Facts:

Serving Size ¼ salad, Calories 202, Fat 6g, Saturated Fat 2g, Cholesterol 5mg, Protein 10g, Carbohydrate 11g, Sugars 5g, Dietary Fiber 2g, Sodium 207mg

Coach Tip

To toast nuts, place them in a small toaster oven on a tray lined with a single layer of foil. Broil the nuts until lightly toasted, about 3 to 5 minutes. Mix them around as they brown to avoid burning. You can use this same procedure for any nut or seed. The smaller the nut or seed the quicker it will cook.

Oriental Beef Salad

An elegant and low-calorie way to have beef as an entrée. Since beef is higher in fat and saturated fat than chicken breast and fish, I recommend, if you want to eat it, have it once a week or less for your health.

YIELD: 4 SERVINGS

MARINADE

1 cup lite teriyaki sauce

¼ cup dry sherry (optional)

2 tablespoons rice wine vinegar

1 teaspoon sesame oil

1 tablespoon honey

2 tablespoons ginger root, minced

1 clove garlic, minced

¼ cup chopped scallion

Juice of ½ a lime

1 teaspoon cayenne

¼ cup cilantro, minced

12 ounces beef sirloin, lean, trimmed of visible fat

SALAD

2 tablespoons sesame seeds

4 cups shredded nappa cabbage

1 cup julienned red pepper

¼ cup sliced scallions, white only

1 cup sliced water chestnuts

1 can mandarin orange slices

1. Mix all the marinade ingredients into a small bowl. Place the meat in a shallow baking dish and pour half the marinade over the sirloin, reserving the other half of the marinade. (If you prefer, you can place the marinade and sirloin into a Ziploc bag and shake to cover with the marinade.) Store in the refrigerator so that the marinade covers the meat.
2. After the steak is marinated, broil or grill the steak until medium-well, about 5 to 7 minutes. You can check the steak by noting when you press down on the steak if it feels like the tip of your nose, tender and not too firm. Once cooked, let the meat rest for 5 minutes and slice into thin slices.
3. While the meat is cooking, broil the sesame seeds in the oven for 2 minutes, until slightly browned.
4. Combine the nappa cabbage, red pepper, scallions, water chestnuts, and mandarin orange slices in a large bowl and mix well. Add the remaining marinade and toss again.

5. Place the sliced meat over the top of the salad, sprinkle with sesame seeds, and serve.

Nutrition Facts:

Serving Size ¼ salad, Calories 180, Fat 6g, Saturated Fat 1g, Cholesterol 51mg, Protein 20g, Carbohydrate 20g, Sugars 10g, Dietary Fiber 4g, Sodium 235mg

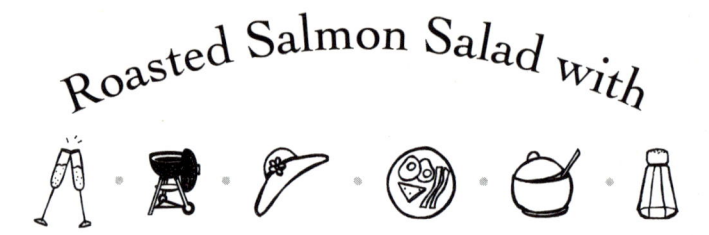

Roasted Salmon Salad with Lemon-Tarragon Buttermilk Dressing

This is a terrific luncheon dish that combines the fresh taste of lemon and tarragon with salmon and asparagus. It will remind you of spring anytime you eat it.

YIELD: 4 SERVINGS

1 pound fresh asparagus

1 red pepper, cut into ⅛-inch slices (or jarred red pepper)

1 pound wild or Pacific salmon filet, cut into 4 portions

1 pound baby spinach leaves

Lemon-Tarragon Buttermilk Dressing (recipe page 112)

Oil spray

1. Prepare the asparagus by cutting off the tough white ends. To make it more tender, you can use a vegetable peeler to peel some layers where it is thick.
2. Place the asparagus on a baking sheet that has been sprayed or lightly brushed with oil spray.

3. On a separate cookie sheet or baking dish, place the red pepper slices skin side up and lightly spray them with oil.
4. Place the salmon filets on a baking sheet lined with aluminum foil.
5. Place the vegetables and the salmon in the oven at 400 degrees to roast. The vegetables will take approximately 10 minutes to roast, the salmon will take about 12 minutes. You will know the vegetables are cooked when they are tender and slightly browned. The salmon should be just cooked through.
6. While the ingredients are roasting, place 2 cups of spinach on each plate.
7. Slice the asparagus into 1-inch pieces. Sprinkle the asparagus and red pepper on top of the spinach.
8. Place the salmon on top of the salad and dress with 3 tablespoons of Lemon-Tarragon Buttermilk Dressing per plate.

Nutrition Facts (per serving) (without dressing):
Serving Size 1/4 *salad, Calories* 220, *Fat* 3g, *Saturated Fat* 1g, *Cholesterol* 59mg, *Protein* 30g, *Carbohydrate* 10g, *Sugars* 3g, *Dietary Fiber* 4g, *Sodium* 105mg

Gayle's Feel-Good Facts

Asparagus is high in folic acid, a vitamin that is helpful for heart health and essential to pregnancy to prevent neural tubal defects. When shopping for asparagus, look for the bright green color, straight firm stalks, and compact tips that are closed and pointed. You can find asparagus steamers that help to cook the asparagus more evenly.

Shrimp with Mango Salsa

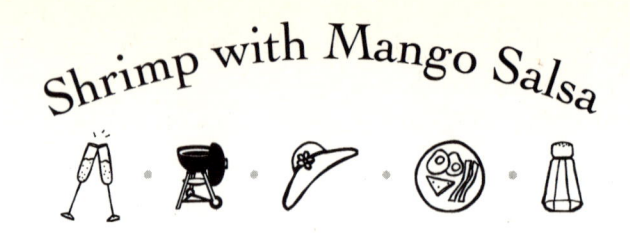

Since shrimp is available all year, you can dine on this light tropical salad anytime and indulge in the flavors of the Carribean.

YIELD: 4 SERVINGS

- 1 red pepper, diced
- 1/4 cup red onion, diced
- 2 mangoes (about 1 cup mango), chopped
- 2 peaches (about 1 cup peaches), chopped
- 1 tablespoon chopped cilantro or 2 teaspoons dry cilantro
- 1/8 cup vegetable broth
- 1/2 small can mild green chilies
- 1 teaspoon white wine vinegar
- Dash of Tabasco (more if you like it spicy)
- 1/8 teaspoon fructose or 1/4 teaspoon sugar
- Juice of 1 lime
- 2 pounds cooked medium shrimp

1. Combine red pepper, onion, mango, peaches, cilantro, broth, chilies, vinegar, Tabasco, fructose, and lime juice in a medium mixing bowl. Stir well to blend.
2. Add the shrimp and serve cold. This dish looks attractive when served in a glass dish or one that has height. It will also look good plated on a bed of salad greens.

■ *Variation*
If peaches are unavailable, you can use pineapple.

Nutrition Facts:
Serving Size 1/4 salad, Calories 108, Fat 1g, Saturated Fat 0g, Cholesterol 147mg, Protein 16g, Carbohydrate 21g, Sugars 21g, Dietary Fiber 3g, Sodium 190mg

Warm Lentil Salad

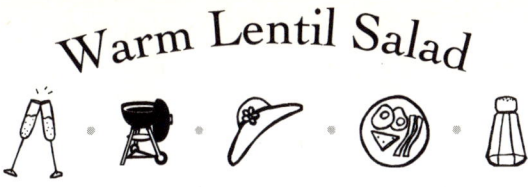

This recipe has evolved based on client requests for a lentil salad. You can use it as a side or put it with greens to make a main course salad for lunch or a light bite.

YIELD: 6 SERVINGS

1 cup dried lentils

¼ cup white wine

1 cup vegetable broth

2 teaspoons Dijon mustard

1 teaspoon chopped thyme

1 tablespoon finely chopped shallots

Juice of 1 lemon

1 tablespoon extra virgin olive oil

¼ teaspoon salt

Pepper to taste

1. Prepare the lentils: Place them in a small saucepan with the white wine and vegetable broth. Bring to a boil, then simmer until the lentils are just cooked, about 20 minutes. When the lentils are firm on the outside and soft on the inside, they are done.
2. In a medium mixing bowl, place the mustard, thyme, shallots, and lemon juice and blend to combine. Then, whisk in the oil so it is well blended.
3. Mix the lentils with the dressing. Add salt and pepper to taste. Serve alone or over mixed greens.

Nutrition Facts:

Serving Size ⅙ salad, *Calories* 72, *Fat* 3g, *Saturated Fat* 0g, *Cholesterol* 0mg, *Protein* 3g, *Carbohydrate* 8g, *Sugars* 1g, *Dietary Fiber* 3g, *Sodium* 307mg

Gayle's Feel-Good Facts

Shallots, onion, leeks, and scallions are all part of the same family as garlic. An ancient symbol of eternity, the onion has sulfur compounds that help to lower blood pressure and quercitin, an antioxidant that defends against cancer and the oxidation of your bad cholesterol (which is what makes the cholesterol stick to your arteries).

Keep onions in a cool dry place to prevent sprouting. To avoid getting tears in your eyes when cutting strong onions, turn on the water and stand by your faucet. This is an old kitchen remedy, but it works.

Dressings

All the dressing listed below can keep for one week in the refrigerator. Aside from using the dressings on salads, they also make great sauces and marinades for fish, chicken, and vegetables. Simply marinate your entrée in the salad dressing for two hours or more. Then grill or roast your entrée. The salad dressing will add flavor to the protein.

Asian Carrot-Ginger Dressing

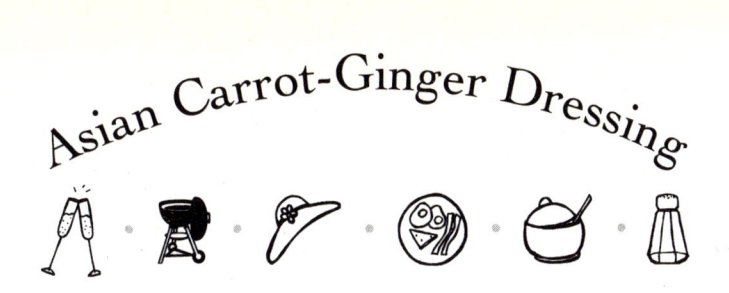

YIELD: 1 CUP

4 carrots, chopped

¼ cup orange juice

2 tablespoons rice wine vinegar

2 tablespoons scallions, minced

2 teaspoons ginger root, minced

¼ teaspoon salt

1 teaspoon freshly ground black pepper

1. In a small pot cover the chopped carrots with water. Bring the water to a boil, lower to simmer, and cook the carrots until soft, approximately 8 minutes.
2. When the carrots are cooked, take them off the heat and drain them.
3. Purée the cooked carrots in a food mill, food processor, or blender.
4. Add the pureed carrots to the remaining ingredients in a large bowl and whisk together.

Nutrition Facts:

Serving Size 2 *tablespoons, Calories* 10, *Fat* 0g, *Saturated Fat* 0g, *Cholesterol* 0mg, *Protein* 0g, *Carbohydrate* 2g, *Sugars* 2g, *Dietary Fiber* 0g, *Sodium* 5mg

Lemon-Tarragon Buttermilk Dressing

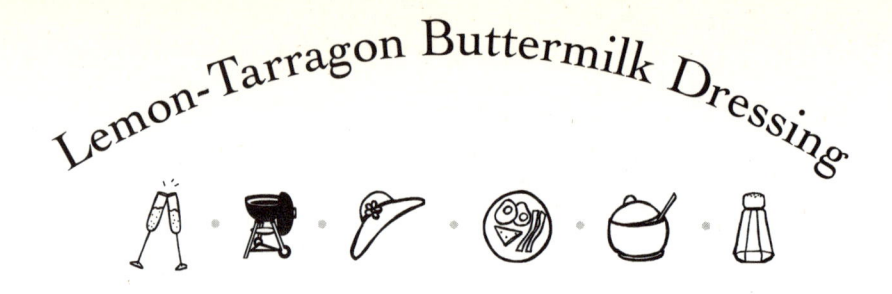

YIELD: 1 CUP

½ cup low-fat buttermilk

1 shallot, minced

½ cup non-fat plain yogurt

Zest of 1 lemon, minced

2 teaspoons minced tarragon or ½ teaspoon dried tarragon

2 teaspoons honey

¼ teaspoon salt

¼ teaspoon freshly ground black pepper

1 tablespoon canola oil

1. Combine all the ingredients together and whisk until well combined. Or, place in a blender or food processor and blend until well combined.
2. Refrigerate until ready to use.

Nutrition Facts:

Serving Size 2 tablespoons, Calories 66, Fat 3g, Saturated Fat 0g, Cholesterol 2mg, Protein 2g, Carbohydrate 8g, Sugars 7g, Dietary Fiber 0g, Sodium 158mg

Gayle's Feel-Good Facts

Although the name implies it comes from butter, buttermilk is actually made by adding bacteria cultures (similar to yogurt) to milk. Look for the low-fat or skim-milk version.

Low-Fat Balsamic Vinaigrette

YIELD: 1 CUP

½ cup fat-free plain yogurt

¼ cup vegetable broth

¼ cup balsamic vinegar

1 shallot, minced

1 clove garlic, minced

1 tablespoon extra virgin olive oil

¼ teaspoon minced thyme or ⅛ teaspoon dried

Pinch of sugar

Pinch of fresh cracked pepper

Pinch of salt

1. Combine the yogurt, broth, vinegar, shallot, and garlic in a medium bowl. Whisk to combine.
2. Add the olive oil and whisk again to combine. Stir in the herbs and seasonings.
3. Refrigerate until ready to use.

Nutrition Facts:

Serving size 2 tablespoons, *Calories* 39, *Fat* 2g, *Saturated Fat* 0g, *Cholesterol* 0mg, *Protein* 0g, *Carbohydrate* 0g, *Sugars* 0g, *Dietary Fiber* 0g, *Sodium* 97mg

Raspberry Vinaigrette

YIELD: 1 CUP

1½ cups fresh or frozen raspberries

¼ teaspoon thyme

¼ teaspoon pepper

3 tablespoons raspberry vinegar

¼ cup water

2 teaspoons canola oil

1½ teaspoons soy sauce

1 tablespoon fructose

1. Combine all the ingredients in a blender and blend until well combined.
2. Refrigerate until ready to use.

Nutrition Facts:

Serving Size 2 tablespoons, *Calories* 6, *Fat* 0g, *Saturated Fat* 0g, *Cholesterol* 0mg, *Protein* 0g, *Carbohydrate* 1g, *Sugars* 0g, *Dietary Fiber* 0g, *Sodium* 16mg

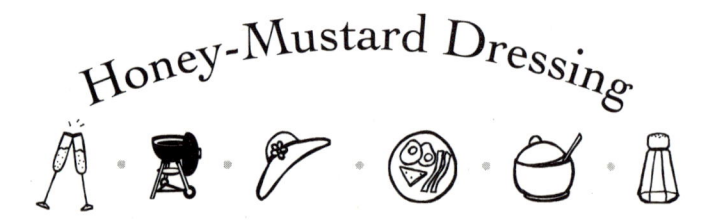

Honey-Mustard Dressing

This dressing keeps for one week, covered in the refrigerator.

YIELD: ½ CUP

½ cup plain nonfat yogurt or soft tofu

¼ cup fresh orange juice

¼ cup rice wine vinegar

2 tablespoons honey

2 tablespoons Dijon mustard

¼ teaspoon ground white pepper

2 teaspoons mustard seed

1. Combine all the ingredients in a blender until smooth.
2. Refrigerate until ready to serve.

Nutrition Facts:

Serving Size 2 tablespoons, *Calories* 50, *Fat* 0g, *Saturated Fat* 0g, *Cholesterol* 0mg, *Protein* 1g, *Carbohydrate* 16g, *Sugars* 10g, *Dietary Fiber* 0g, *Sodium* 160mg

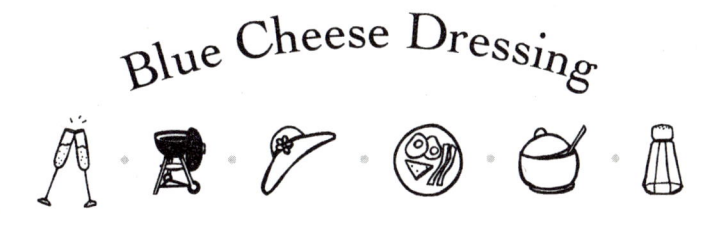

Blue Cheese Dressing

YIELD: 1 ½ CUPS

¾ cup low-fat buttermilk

⅓ cup fat-free mayonnaise

½ teaspoon minced garlic (1 clove)

¼ cup crumbled blue cheese

2 ½ tablespoons nonfat cottage cheese

1. In a blender combine the buttermilk, mayonnaise, and garlic. Blend until smooth.
2. Transfer to a medium bowl. Stir in the blue cheese and cottage cheese. Chill until ready to serve.

Nutrition Facts:

Serving Size 2 tablespoons, *Calories* 46, *Fat* 2g, *Saturated Fat* 1g, *Cholesterol* 6mg, *Protein* 3g, *Carbohydrate* 3g, *Sugars* 2g, *Dietary Fiber* 0g, *Sodium* 225mg

Fresh Herb Vinaigrette

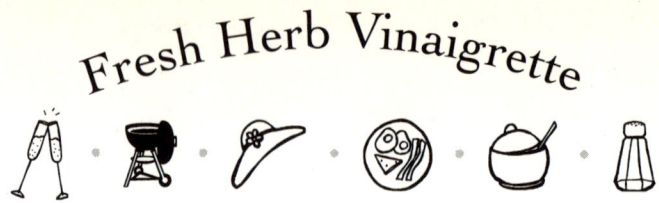

YIELD: 2 CUPS (8 SERVINGS)

½ cup red wine vinegar

¼ teaspoon black pepper

2 cloves garlic, minced

1 tablespoon Dijon mustard

Juice of ½ lemon

½ teaspoon salt

1 tablespoon fructose

2 teaspoons Worcestershire

1 tablespoon chopped basil

¾ cup water or broth

1. Combine all the ingredients except water in a blender and blend. Add the water or broth. Blend again.
2. Refrigerate until ready to use.

Nutrition Facts:

Serving Size 2 tablespoons, *Calories* 10, *Fat* 0g, *Saturated Fat* 0g, *Cholesterol* 0mg, *Protein* 0g, *Carbohydrate* 2g, *Sugars* 1g, *Dietary Fiber* 0g, *Sodium* 208mg

Low-Fat Caesar Salad Dressing

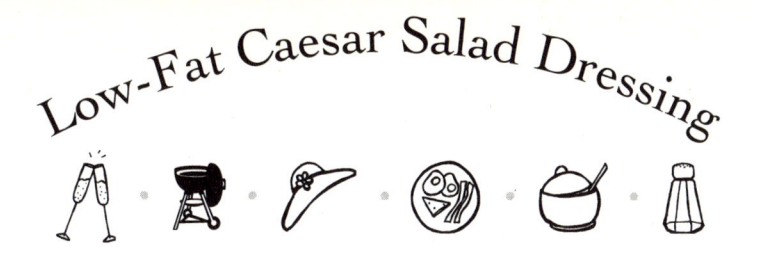

YIELD: ¾ CUP

WILL KEEP FOR ONE WEEK COVERED IN THE REFRIGERATOR.

½ cup (8 fl oz/125 ml) plain nonfat yogurt

2 tablespoons grated Parmesan

1 tablespoon fresh lemon juice

1 teaspoon Worcestershire Sauce

1 teaspoon Dijon mustard

2 whole Anchovies or 1 teaspoon Anchovy paste

½ teaspoon black pepper

1 clove garlic, mashed or chopped finely

Pinch of cayenne pepper

Salt, to taste

1. Combine all the ingredients in a blender until smooth; adjust seasoning to taste with salt and pepper. Refrigerate until ready to use.

Nutrition Facts:

Calories 22, Fat 1g, Saturated Fat 0g, Cholesterol 2mg, Protein 2g, Carbohydrate 2g, Sugars 2g, Dietary Fiber 0g, Sodium 87mg

6

Sandwiches

There is nothing like sinking your teeth into a great-tasting sandwich. Not only is it a fun eating experience, but sandwiches afford you the opportunity to indulge in a combination of delicious tastes all in one bite. Unfortunately, I find that many people avoid sandwiches when they are watching their weight because the perception is that they are fattening and high in carbs. Sandwiches, while they have two pieces of bread, are often the same calorie content as a salad, and sometimes they have even less calories than a salad, because the salad dressing really can add up calorically. Since a sandwich is sometimes more filling than a salad and often has the same number of calories, it is sometimes the better lunch choice if you are trying to cut back on snacking and are watching your weight. Sandwiches are even a great option for a light dinner.

I have included some tasty combinations that are sure to tempt you. Plus, there is a section on making salads into sandwiches, such as wraps or pita sandwiches. This is easy to do. When you are on the go, packing a sandwich is easier than packing a salad.

BBQ Baked Tofu and Vegetable Wrap

Even if tofu doesn't appeal to you, you will like this sandwich. The sweet taste of the BBQ sauce and the crunchy vegetables complement each other so well, you won't miss the meat.

YIELD: 1 WRAP

1 4-ounce square tofu lin (or very firm tofu)

¼ cup BBQ Sauce (page 152 or purchase premade)

1 10-inch whole-wheat flour tortilla or wrap bread

1 carrot, sliced thin

¼ cup sweet corn

¼ cup zucchini, sliced thin

1 scallion, white only, sliced thin

¼ cup baby spinach leaves

¼ cup alfalfa sprouts

1. Slice the tofu into ¼-inch thin slices.
2. Place the tofu on a nonstick or foil-lined baking sheet. Coat with BBQ sauce and bake for 10 minutes. BBQ sauce is well cooked onto tofu.
3. Lay the bread on a flat service, such as a cutting board. Lay all the ingredients in the center of the wrap bread so they lay flat.
4. Fold the wrap as follows: Fold in the sides first, then roll the bread with filling in it from the top to the bottom. Lay the sandwich on the cutting board so that the bottom seam of the bread is on the bottom. Cut in half on the diagonal and serve.

Nutrition Facts:

Serving Size 1 sandwich, Calories 440, Fat 13g, Saturated Fat 2g, Cholesterol 0mg, Protein 28g, Carbohydrate 60g, Sugars 23g, Dietary Fiber 16g, Sodium 1130mg

Curry Chicken with Apples in Pita

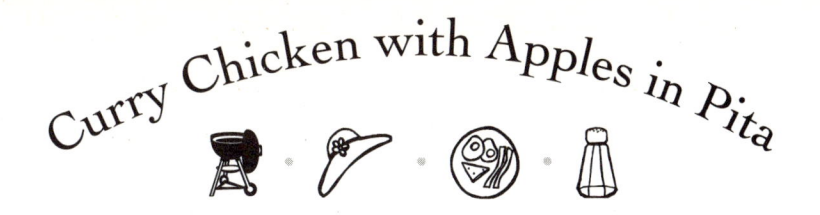

The curry and apples combine to give you spicy and sweet tastes, plus the fruit and vegetables provide a satisfying crunch with every bite.

YIELD: 1 SANDWICH

FILLING

1 3-ounce chicken breast

¼ Granny Smith apple, sliced thin

½ celery stalk, sliced thin

5 grapes, sliced in half

1 romaine lettuce leaf, shredded

2 teaspoons curry powder

¼ teaspoon cumin

⅛ teaspoon salt

Pinch cayenne

1 large whole-wheat pita

CURRY YOGURT SAUCE

¾ cup tomato paste

⅓ cup nonfat plain yogurt

1. Grill or broil the chicken until cooked, about 10 minutes. When finished, slice in chunks.
2. Mix the apples, celery, and grapes together in a medium bowl and set aside.
3. To make the sauce, place all the sauce ingredients in a blender or food processor and blend until smooth.
4. Slice a ¼ inch off the top of the pita, so you can open it up and stuff it.
5. Place 2 tablespoons of the sauce inside the pita and spread it around.
6. Stuff the pita with the lettuce, then sprinkle in the chicken and apple mixture.

7. Top with 1 tablespoon of the dressing. Reserve the remainder of the sauce to use as a vegetable dip or on additional sandwiches.

Nutrition Facts:
Serving Size 1 sandwich, *Calories* 590, *Fat* 11g, *Saturated Fat* 3g, *Cholesterol* 55mg, *Protein* 35g, *Carbohydrate* 100g, *Sugars* 28g, *Dietary Fiber* 17g, *Sodium* 900mg

Gayle's Feel-Good Facts

Yogurt is a great ingredient in low-fat recipes because it adds a thickness and creamy quality to sauces, while still fat-free and healthy. Yogurt is packed with calcium and contains live bacteria cultures, which help keep your intestines healthy and digestion working well.

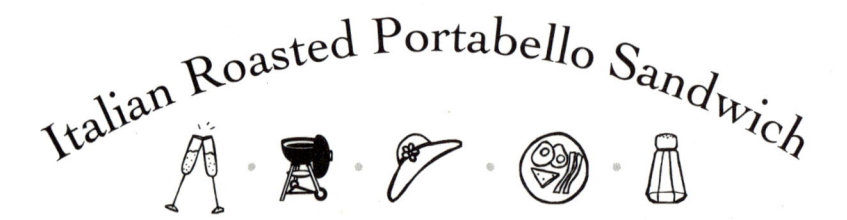

Italian Roasted Portabello Sandwich

When you are in need of something meaty to sink your teeth into but don't want to eat beef, try a portabello mushroom. They have a similar firm texture and meaty-mushroom flavor.

YIELD: 1 SANDWICH

1 portabello mushroom

Oil spray

2 tablespoons sundried tomato paste

2 ounces low-fat goat cheese

2 slices whole-grain bread

½ cup baby spinach leaves

½ roasted red pepper

1 sliced tomato

1. Roast a whole portabello mushroom. To roast, oil a nonstick or foiled-lined baking dish with oil spray. Place the portabello mushroom in a baking dish and roast at 400 degrees for 8 to 10 minutes, or until soft and cooked.
2. Mix the sundried tomato paste with the goat cheese in a small bowl and spread on one side of each slice of bread. Layer the portabella, baby spinach leaves, roasted red pepper, and tomato between the slices of bread. Serve.

Nutrition Facts:

Serving Size 1 sandwich, *Calories* 210, *Fat* 7g, *Saturated Fat* 3g, *Cholesterol* 15mg, *Protein* 14g, *Carbohydrate* 27g, *Sugars* 3g, *Dietary Fiber* 7g, *Sodium* 530mg

Gayle's Feel-Good Facts

Many people who have a dairy allergy are actually allergic to the protein in cow's milk products. The protein found in goat and sheep milk is similar to that of a cow, but not the same. Therefore, most adults with a dairy allergy can tolerate cheeses made from goat and sheep milk, but these cheeses are not recommended for infants and children.

Mixed Bean, Vegetable, and Cheese Quesadilla

A fast and healthy way to make a tasty lunch. This is also a fun recipe to make with a group or family.

YIELD: 4 SERVINGS

8 6-inch whole-wheat or corn tortillas

1 cup black beans, drained and rinsed

1 cup frozen corn, thawed

1 cup low-fat cheddar cheese

4 plum tomatoes, diced

4 scallions, sliced

½ cup cilantro, chopped

1 pound fat-free sour cream

8 ounces Avocado Tomatillo (recipe page 57) or pre-made tomato salsa

Oil spray

1. Preheat the oven to 325 degrees. Spray a baking sheet with oil or brush with oil.
2. Place the tortillas on the baking sheet and cook in the oven for 3 minutes. Remove from the oven and turn the tortillas over on the tray to fill.
3. In a separate bowl, mix the black beans and corn and spread evenly on the tortillas.
4. Sprinkle cheese over the bean and corn mixture and lay the second tortilla on top.
5. Bake in the oven for 10 minutes. In the last 1 to 2 minutes broil the tortilla to get the top light brown and toasted.
6. Serve with chopped tomato, scallion, cilantro, sour cream, and tomatilla on the side.

Nutrition Facts:

Serving Size 1 quesadilla, Calories 400, Fat 5g, Saturated Fat 1g, Cholesterol 15mg, Protein 27g, Carbohydrate 61g, Sugars 13g, Dietary Fiber 15g, Sodium 620mg

Roasted Vegetable Sandwich with Hummus

Getting veggies into your daily diet is not always easy. By using roasted vegetables on a sandwich with a spread, it becomes easy to pack in taste and health for a quick meal.

YIELD: 4 SANDWICHES

GRILLED VEGETABLES

2 red peppers

1 small eggplant

1 1/3 zucchini

2/3 cup Low-Fat Balsamic Vinaigrette (page 113)

2/3 cup mushrooms

1 leek

HUMMUS (for recipe see pg 59)

1 loaf Italian whole-wheat bread

1/4 pound arugula

1. Place the peppers on a baking sheet and roast at 400 degrees until all sides are black and charred. Take out of the oven and cover with a paper bag or plastic wrap. When cool, peel the skins off, core, and deseed. Slice and put aside.
2. Slice the eggplant and zucchini lengthwise up to 1/4 inch thick. Toss in 1/3 cup vinaigrette and place on baking sheet. Roast at 450 degrees until soft. Remove and cool.
3. Slice the mushrooms and leeks. Toss in 1/3 cup vinaigrette and sauté in Teflon pan until tender, or roast in oven.
4. Prepare the hummus as directed by the recipe on page 59.
5. Slice the bread lengthwise three-quarters way through; leaving one side attached. Remove the inside bread from the bottom part of the loaf. Spread the hummus on the bottom. Layer the vegetables, top with arugula, and serve.

Nutrition Facts:

Serving Size 1 sandwich, Calories 254, Fat 6g, Saturated Fat 0g, Cholesterol 0mg, Protein 12g, Carbohydrate 45g, Sugars 9g, Dietary Fiber 11g, Sodium 181mg

Gayle's Feel-Good Facts

Arugula is not just a fancy lettuce: It is actually a cruciferous vegetable, which means it has cancer-fighting nutrients and is packed with vitamin C. It has a somewhat bitter taste, so it is good to pair it with other flavors or mix it with other greens for a salad.

Suggested Wrap Combinations for Sandwiches

Wrap sandwiches are very popular and easy to make. The best sandwiches are those that have interesting ingredients combined together. Below I have listed how to turn some common salads into wraps, as well as additional options for making simple wrap sandwiches. When you are on the go, packing a wrap can make life a bit easier than packing a salad.

To make a wrap: Use a 10- to 12-inch tortilla or wrap bread, place the ingredients in the center of the tortilla or wrap bread to form a small flat mound. Fold the sides of the tortilla into the center and then roll up the tortilla from the top to the bottom. Serve by cutting the wrap in half on a diagonal in the center with the seam on the bottom.

OPTIONAL FILLINGS

For each wrap, either divide the salad recipe into the number of servings listed in the recipe or, use 3 ounces of fish, meat, or chicken per wrap, several slices of tomato, $\frac{1}{4}$ to $\frac{1}{2}$ cup of salad greens, and a pinch of any additional vegetable (peppers, cucumbers, etc). When slicing vegetables for wraps, it is ideal to either slice them in thin strips or slices, so when you eat the sandwich you get some with each bite.

- Broiled salmon, 2 tablespoons of Honey Mustard Dressing (page 114), sliced tomato, mesclun greens, sliced red pepper, and sliced cucumber
- Smoked salmon, capers, mustard, and baby spinach leaves
- Chicken or turkey breast, 2 tablespoons BBQ Sauce (page 152), mesclun, tomatoes, cucumber, carrots
- Low-fat mozzarella, 2 tablespoons pesto sauce, tomatoes, and shredded green leaf lettuce
- Chicken breast, 2 tablespoons red pepper aioli (page 56), green leaf lettuce, sliced artichoke hearts, and chopped sundried tomatoes.

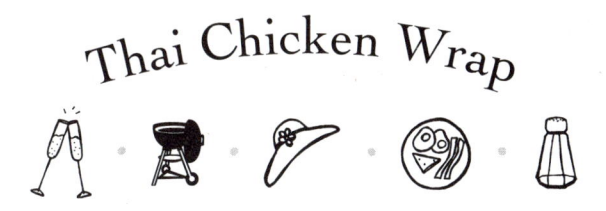

Thai Chicken Wrap

The Thai marinade provides an easy and excellent way to spice up a traditional chicken sandwich. You can refrigerate the marinade in an airtight container for up to one week.

YIELD: 1 SANDWICH

THAI MARINADE

1 cup lite coconut milk

1 cup chopped cilantro

1 tablespoon curry powder

¼ teaspoon turmeric

1 serrano or one jalepeno chili, seeded and chopped

2 tablespoons fructose

1 clove garlic

1 teaspoon chopped ginger

1 tablespoon fresh lime juice

1 tablespoon canola or peanut oil

FILLING

1 grilled or broiled chicken breast

1 10-inch whole-wheat tortilla or wrap bread

½ cup Boston or bibb lettuce, shredded

¼ cup julienned cucumbers

¼ cup shredded carrot

¼ cup julienned red pepper

2 basil leaves, julienned

1. Combine all the ingredients for the marinade except the oil, in a blender. Blend until smooth. Pour into a bowl, add the oil, and mix well. Marinate the chicken breast in ¼ cup of the Thai marinade for 1 hour or more before cooking.
2. Broil or grill the marinaded chicken breast on medium heat until cooked through, about 10 minutes. Remove from the heat and let cool to room temperature.
3. Lay the tortilla or wrap bread on a dry cutting board. Sprinkle the lettuce, cucumber, red pepper, and basil around the center of the bread.
4. Slice the chicken breast into strips. Lay the strips in the center of the bread. Sprinkle with 2 tablespoons of Thai Marinade. Make sure the wrap ingredients are lying flat and not too mounded in the center of the bread.
5. Fold up the wrap as follows: Turn the sides of the wrap in and then from the top of the wrap roll the sandwich toward you.

Nutrition Facts:

Serving Size 1 sandwich, Calories 270, Fat 9g, Saturated Fat 2g, Cholesterol 70mg, Protein 28g, Carbohydrate 16g, Sugars 7g, Dietary Fiber 4g, Sodium 85mg

7

Entrées

The recipes listed in this section are intended to help you answer that age-old question, "What's for dinner?" Some recipes are more elaborate than others and can be used for entertaining and company, while others are quick and easy and intended to take twenty minutes or less to prepare. So that you don't have to give up your favorite foods while eating healthy, many recipes are light versions of traditional family favorites: There really is no reason to have to forgo a meal you want. It just needs to be made in a slightly different manner.

Taste, as always, is the reason a recipe made it into this book. Even though a meal is low-fat, you should still be able to sit down and savor every bite and treat yourself to a delicious eating experience. Of course, the fresher your ingredients, the better tasting your meal, but if you are short on time you can reduce your prep time by using ingredients that are already semi-prepped for you at your local supermarket.

I have provided you with quick tips for adding flavor to meat, fish, and poultry, as well as more elaborate vegetarian, meat, poultry, fish, and seafood recipes. Aside from the quick twenty minute or less recipes, many of the entrées can be made ahead and frozen, so that you can be well prepared with healthy meals for those times when you don't have the opportunity to cook.

Techniques and Tricks to Quickly Cook an Entrée That Is Packed with Flavor

When it comes time to make dinner, many people want to spend as little time in the kitchen as possible. There are many fast ways to add flavor to a basic broiled, grilled, or baked chicken breast, fish, steak, or filet. Below are two simple steps to whip up a delightful, tasty repast in twenty minutes or less.

STEP 1—USE HERB AND SPICE BLENDS TO ENHANCE FLAVOR

Make sure you have some of these items in the refrigerator and pantry at all times for those spur-of-the-moment meals:

- **Bottled Marinades**: You can find these in your local supermarket or gourmet store. Choose the ones that sound appealing to you. Finding your favorites will be a bit of trial and error. Most bottled marinades are fat-free. If you want to make sure the sauce you choose is healthy, look to see that it has 3 grams of fat or less. If you are watching your sodium, the sauce should also have 400 mg of sodium or less. You can also make marinades from the salad dressing recipes in chapter 5 or any of the marinades listed in this book.
- **Tapenades and Pestos**: A tapenade is traditionally a purée of olives in olive oil, but these days you can also find sundried tomato tapenades as well as many others. Pesto is a thick Italian sauce typically made of a blend of basil,

olive oil, pine nuts, and Parmesan cheese. While you can find many basil pestos at your market, also look for artichoke pesto and others that sound appealing. Both tapenades and pestos make excellent spreads and coatings on fish. Refer to the recipes for Quick and Light Pesto and Sundried Tomato–Roasted Red Pepper Tapanade in this chapter.

If you would like to add herbs to your cooking, refer to the herb chart on page 21. Recipes in this book that you can have on hand for this purpose include the Artichoke Dip recipe on page 55 and the Eggplant Caviar recipe on page 66.

Quick and Light Pesto

YIELD: 6 SERVINGS

4 cups chopped and packed fresh basil leaves

½ cup vegetable broth

¼ cup pine nuts or walnuts

3 tablespoons extra virgin olive oil

½ teaspoon salt

3 garlic cloves, peeled

¼ cup grated fresh Parmesan Reggiano cheese

Combine all the ingredients in a food processor; process until finely minced. If you like a thinner sauce, add more broth. This can keep in the refrigerator for a week or freezer for 3 months.

Nutrition Facts:

Serving Size ¼ cup, Calories 313, Fat 12g, Saturated Fat 1g, Cholesterol 3mg, Protein 20g, Carbohydrate 32g, Sugars 0g, Dietary Fiber 25g, Sodium 347mg

Sundried Tomato–Roasted Red Pepper Tapenade

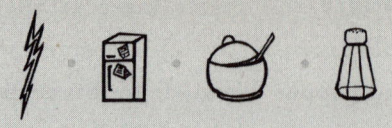

YIELD: 16-1 TABLESPOON SERVINGS

3 large, firm red bell peppers, roasted and peeled, or jarred in oil

3/4 cup sundried tomatoes, soaked in hot water for 15 minutes to reconstitute

1 clove of garlic, peeled

2 tablespoons extra virgin olive oil

1/4 teaspoon salt

1/2 teaspoon black pepper

Dash of red pepper flakes (optional)

Combine all the ingredients in a food processor; process until finely minced. This can keep in the refrigerator for a week or freezer for 3 months.

Nutrition Facts:

Serving Size 1 tablespoon, *Calories* 29, *Fat* 2g, *Saturated Fat* 0g, *Cholesterol* 0mg, *Protein* 0g, *Carbohydrate* 3g, *Sugars* 1g, *Dietary Fiber* 1g, *Sodium* 90mg

- **Flavorful spreads and low-fat mayonnaise**: Since low-fat mayonnaise is a good way to moisten foods, blending it with flavor and spreading it on fish or chicken is an easy way to dress up any meal. Try experimenting with Grey Poupon mustard, wasabi powder (Asian mustard powder), or miso paste (the white miso) mixed with low-fat mayonnaise. Add herb mixtures to the mayonnaise base to achieve a variety of fresh flavors:
    - Grey Poupon mayonnaise with herbs de Provence or bouquet garni herb blends
    - Wasabi mayonnaise with sesame seeds, a dash of ginger, or dried onions
    - Miso mayonnaise with sesame seeds, a dash of soy sauce, or a splash of mirin (Asian cooking wine)

- **Spice Rubs**: In the spice aisle of your market you will find many different spice rubs that are already combined to be used with chicken, fish, or meat. While these do not add moisture, they do add quite a bit of flavor. A good way to cook with them is to sprinkle the seasoning on your chicken or fish, wrap it in foil to maintain moisture, and cook. See step 2 for roasting directions.

Step 2—Roast to Perfection

Preheat the oven to 350 degrees or heat the grill (an indoor grill is good to use as well) and coat the fish or chicken breast with your flavor-enhancing blend of choice. Keep extra sauce available so you can baste the main entrée midway through cooking. Following are roasting instructions for specific foods:

- Fish: For thin fish, roast in the oven for three to five minutes per side. For meatier fish like salmon, roast for ten minutes per inch.
- Chicken or turkey breast: Roast for ten to twelve minutes. For lean meats, use marinades and broil to desired doneness: medium takes about ten minutes. You can check if meat is cooked to medium by comparing the meat to the tip of your nose. If it feels the same in terms of how firm it is, then you have cooked the meat to medium, medium-rare. If the meat is softer, it is rare; if the meat is more firm, chances are good that you have cooked the meat to medium-well or well.

VEGETARIAN ENTRÉES

BBQ Beans and Tofu

Instead of tofu, you can use vegetarian "hot dogs" for a healthy version of a "pork and beans" recipe.

YIELD: 6 SERVINGS

1 teaspoon canola oil	1 teaspoon Tabasco
2 garlic cloves, minced	1 teaspoon dried thyme
1 cup finely chopped onion	1 bay leaf
2 cups navy beans from can, drained	1 whole clove
1 cup BBQ Sauce (page 152, or buy premade)	¼ teaspoon salt
¼ cup Dijon mustard	Pepper
½ cup maple syrup	1 pound baked tofu cut into 1-inch chunks, or tofu lin (Note: The baked tofu can have a marinade if it is not available plain)

1. In a large pot, add the oil and gently cook the garlic and onion over low heat until translucent, then stir in the beans to combine. Turn off the heat and set aside.
2. Combine the BBQ sauce, mustard, maple syrup, Tabasco, thyme, bay leaf, clove, salt, and pepper.
3. Stir the sauce in with the tofu. Add the bean mixture to the tofu mixture in a medium-large mixing bowl.
4. Place the tofu-bean mixture in an 8-x-8-inch baking dish. Cover and bake at 350 degrees for 30 minutes, stirring once during the baking.
5. When well heated, serve hot.

Nutrition Facts:

Serving Size 1 cup, Calories 245, Fat 2g, Saturated Fat 0g, Cholesterol 0mg, Protein 6g, Carbohydrate 52g, Sugars 31g, Dietary Fiber 5g, Sodium 972mg

Black Bean and Spinach Burritos

These are a real crowd pleaser for family and friends, because they taste so fresh and are packed with healthy vegetables and low-fat cheese. They can be frozen and keep for up to a month.

YIELD: 6 SERVINGS

BEANS

1 teaspoon canola oil

1 onion, diced

1 green bell pepper, diced

2 tablespoons fresh orange juice

2 cloves garlic, minced

1 teaspoon ground cumin

½ teaspoon chili powder

1 teaspoon adobo chili seasoning (optional)

1 cup chopped canned plum tomatoes with juice

2 15-ounce cans black beans, drained

2 tablespoons fresh lime juice

2 tablespoons chopped cilantro

Pinch of sugar or fructose

RICE

1 cup brown rice

1 teaspoon ground cumin

½ teaspoon turmeric

2 cups water

½ teaspoon salt

TORTILLA

2 pounds fresh spinach, washed, stemmed, and cleaned

6 large low-fat whole-wheat tortillas (12 inches in diameter)

1½ cups grated low-fat cheddar or soy cheddar cheese

1. For the beans, heat a large saucepan over high heat until very hot. Add the oil followed by the onion and sear for 30 seconds.
2. Add the peppers and sear for 30 seconds.

3. Add the orange juice to deglaze and stir well.
4. Add the garlic, turn down the heat to medium, and add the cumin and chili and adobo powders. Stir vigorously for 15 seconds to release the flavors. Stir in the tomatoes with their juice. Cook for 2 minutes.
5. Add the black beans and lime juice, stir gently, and add water halfway up the saucepan. Cook over low heat, uncovered, until the liquid is thick, about 15 minutes. Add the cilantro and season to taste. An extra squeeze of lime juice or pinch of sugar or fructose can be added to taste.
6. Put the rice, cumin, and turmeric in a saucepan. Add the water and bring to a boil, uncovered, and turn down the heat.
7. Cook, uncovered, over low heat for 30 to 40 minutes, or until the liquid has been absorbed. Fluff the rice with a fork and season with salt.
8. Place the cleaned spinach with the water still clinging to its leaves in a hot skillet and cook until just wilted.
9. Let cool and squeeze out excess moisture.
10. Lay the tortilla on a work surface. Place ¼ cup cooked rice, a generous ½ cup beans, ¼ cup spinach, and 2 tablespoons cheese on the bottom end of the tortilla. Fold over sides, then roll up. Serve.
11. The burritos can also be sealed in an airtight bag and frozen. Burritos can be reheated in a microwave or warmed seam side down, wrapped in foil, in a 325 degree oven for 10 minutes.

Nutrition Facts:

Serving Size 1 burrito, *Calories* 442, *Fat* 7g, *Saturated Fat* 1g, *Cholesterol* 6mg, *Protein* 32g, *Carbohydrate* 68g, *Sugars* 7g, *Dietary Fiber* 24g, *Sodium* 617mg

Sundried Tomato and Basil Sauce

This is an all-purpose sauce that freezes beautifully and can be used in various pasta recipes, but it also works great as a base for other dishes.

YIELD: 18 SERVINGS

1 cup chopped sundried tomatoes (not in oil)

1 cup vegetable broth

1 28-ounce can plum tomatoes

1 medium onion, finely diced

4 cloves garlic chopped

1 teaspoon olive oil

1 28-ounce can crushed tomatoes in purée

½ cup dry red wine

2 bay leaves

2 whole cloves

½ teaspoon crushed red pepper

½ teaspoon dried oregano

1 teaspoon brown sugar

1 cup fresh basil chiffonade

¼ teaspoon fresh parsley

1. Rehydrate the sundried tomatoes by simmering them in the vegetable broth in a small sauce pot. When they are very soft, remove them from the broth, about 15 minutes. Save the infused broth.
2. Coarsely blend tomatoes in a food processor. Set aside.
3. Purée the plum tomatoes in a blender or food processor. Set aside.
4. Sweat the onion and garlic in oil in a heavy broth pot. Add the infused vegetable broth and sweat until the onion is soft.
5. Add the puréed tomatoes, crushed tomatoes, sundried tomato mixture, red wine, bay leaves, cloves, red pepper, oregano, and brown sugar.
6. Simmer for 20 minutes, until flavors are well blended. Stir in chopped basil and parsley. Use as desired or store in a container in the freezer for later use.

Nutrition Facts:

Serving Size ½ cup, Calories 31, Fat 0g, Saturated Fat 0g, Cholesterol 0mg, Protein 1g, Carbohydrate 5g, Sugars 3g, Dietary Fiber 1g, Sodium 188mg

Baked Ziti with Vegetables

The seasonings give this common dish a special flavor. Plus you can have a traditional Italian favorite without the guilt of the high-fat cheese. This is a great comfort food meal on a cold day.

YIELD: 8 TO 10 SERVINGS

1 small onion, chopped

2 cloves garlic, minced

2 teaspoons olive oil

½ cup red wine

4 cups chopped tomatoes

1 pound whole-wheat ziti

1 pound spinach or swiss chard

1 tablespoon balsamic vinegar

1 cup skim-milk ricotta

½ cup Parmesan cheese

3 tablespoons chopped basil

3 tablespoons chopped Italian parsley

1 teaspoon oregano

½ pound grated part-skim mozzarella

Oil spray or oil for coating baking dish

1. In a large saucepan, sauté the onion and garlic in 2 teaspoons of olive oil. Add the wine and tomatoes. Simmer until slightly thick, about 30 minutes.
2. Cook the ziti as directed on the package while preparing the spinach-cheese mixture. Clean the spinach or chard and chop roughly. In a large soup pot

cook the spinach in 1 teaspoon of oil until wilted. Add the vinegar, ricotta, ½ cup Parmesan cheese, basil, parsley, and oregano to greens and set aside.

3. Combine tomatoes with ziti and cheese mixture. Spray or lightly oil baking dish. Pour ziti mixture into the dish to bake.
4. Sprinkle the mozzarella and remaining Parmesan on top of the ziti. Bake at 350 degrees for 30 minutes. Serve hot.

Nutrition Facts:

Serving Size 1½ cups, Calories 349, Fat 9g, Saturated Fat 4g, Cholesterol 65mg, Protein 23g, Carbohydrate 42g, Sugars 8g, Dietary Fiber 5g, Sodium 435mg

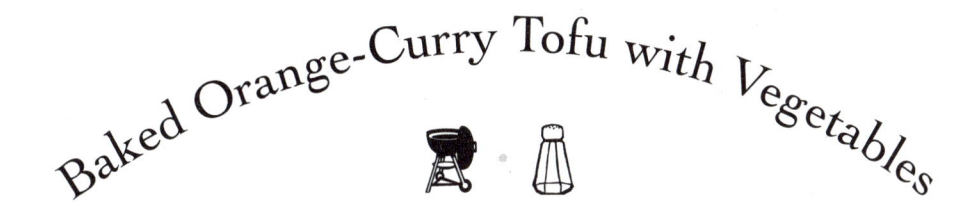

Baked Orange-Curry Tofu with Vegetables

Easy to make and serve, this sweet recipe for tofu is a satisfying blend of flavors and textures.

YIELD: 4 SKEWERS

MARINADE

2 teaspoons honey

1 tablespoon curry powder

¼ cup orange juice

1 teaspoon cumin

¼ cup vegetable broth

1 teaspoon chopped basil

1 teaspoon chopped cilantro

1 teaspoon minced garlic

1 teaspoon minced ginger

TOFU AND VEGETABLES

4 large bamboo or metal skewers (optional)

1 zucchini, sliced in ½-inch rounds

8 large whole mushrooms

4 large pineapple chunks

8 slices red or yellow pepper (1 large pepper)

4 slices red onion

16 cubes 1 inch x 1 inch tofu lin (baked tofu) or extra firm tofu

2 cups cooked brown rice

1. Combine all the marinade ingredients in a small mixing bowl.
2. *Skewer the above ingredients in the following order, either on metal or bamboo skewers: zucchini, a mushroom, a pineapple chunk, a pepper slice, an onion slice, and a cube of tofu. Repeat until the skewer is finished. (*Soak the bamboo skewers, make sure you soak them in water first for 20 to 30 minutes.) If you do not use skewers, soak the vegetables and tofu in the sauce in a medium-large mixing bowl.
3. Place the skewers in a baking dish and pour the marinade over the skewers. Allow to marinate for an hour or more.
4. Grill or broil until cooked, about 5 minutes. If not using skewers, sauté vegetables and tofu in sauce until cooked, about 8 to 10 minutes.
5. Serve the skewers or sautéed tofu and vegetables over the brown rice.

Nutrition Facts:

Serving Size 1 large skewer, and ½ cup of rice, *Calories* 198, *Fat* 3g, *Saturated Fat* 0g, *Cholesterol* 0mg, *Protein* 10g, *Carbohydrate* 35g, *Sugars* 9g, *Dietary Fiber* 4g, *Sodium* 60mg

Gayle's Feel-Good Facts

Tofu, soybeans, and soy milk are all from the same bean, the soybean. Soy is a very versatile bean because it has a very mild flavor. It can take on most flavors that you mix it with. It also has about twice the amount of protein ounce for ounce when compared to other beans. Plus, the soybean contains protective antioxidants called isoflavones, which help prevent some hormone-dependent cancers (breast, prostate), and bolster bones, and the protein in soy assists in lowering low-density lipoproteins ("bad" LDL cholesterol).

Soy Moo Shu

Easier to make than it sounds, this traditional Chinese dish will impress all those who eat it. You can also make this a chicken or shrimp moo shu by substituting or adding one pound of chicken or shrimp to the recipe instead of, or in addition to, the tofu.

YIELD: 8 SERVINGS

SAUCE

¼ cup low-sodium soy

⅓ cup Mirin

1 tablespoon hoisin sauce

1 tablespoon cornstarch dissolved in 3 tablespoons water

TOFU

4 cups tofu lin (available at health-food stores) or baked tofu

½ cup orange juice

4 cups spinach, cleaned and shredded, or 4 cups baby spinach leaves

4 cups julienned nappa cabbage

4 cups sliced shitake mushrooms

3 cups julienned leeks (approximately 3 leeks)

3 cups julienned carrots (approximately 6 large carrots)

2 cups julienned red bell pepper (approximately 2 large peppers)

6 cloves garlic, minced

2 tablespoons minced ginger (about 2 inches in length if using fresh)

1 teaspoon canola oil

8 teaspoons hoisin sauce, served on the side

8 moo shu pancakes or whole-wheat tortillas

1. Prepare the moo shu sauce by placing all the ingredients in a small bowl and whisking to combine. Set aside.
2. Slice the tofu into $\frac{1}{4}$-inch slices and place in the bowl with the orange juice. Let marinade while you prepare the remainder of the recipe.
3. Combine all the vegetables, garlic, and ginger and set aside.
4. Heat a wok or sauté pan with 1 teaspoon canola oil on high for 3 minutes, or until the pan is very hot. Be careful that the oil does not begin smoking. If it does, turn the heat down.
5. Drain the tofu mixture and combine with the vegetable mixture. Place in the hot pan and stir briskly.
6. When the vegetables are barely cooked, add the moo shu sauce. Mix thoroughly until the sauce thickens. Remove from the heat.
7. Serve with moo shu pancakes or tortillas, with sauce on the side or mix hoisin sauce with brown rice and top with moo shu vegetables and tofu.

Variation

Asian and health-food stores sell soy chicken that you can use instead of tofu in this recipe.

Nutrition Facts:

Serving Size 1 pancake or $\frac{1}{8}$ of mixture, Calories 289, Fat 6g, Saturated Fat 0g, Cholesterol 0mg, Protein 18g, Carbohydrate 39g, Sugars 10g, Dietary Fiber 11g, Sodium 620mg

Gayle's Feel-Good Facts

Hot pepper sauce not only adds a kick to your foods, but it also punches up your immune system, acts as a digestive aid, and stimulates circulation.

Spinach and Ricotta Stuffed Shells

The low-fat cheese combined with the seasoning makes this a satisfying and tasty way to have a comforting meal that is typically high fat.

YIELD: 6 SERVINGS

12 jumbo pasta shells, whole-wheat if possible

½ onion, chopped

2 cloves garlic, chopped fine

½ pound part-skim or low-fat ricotta cheese

½ pound baby spinach, trimmed, washed, chopped

¼ cup grated Parmesan cheese

Black pepper to taste

⅛ teaspoon nutmeg

¼ teaspoon salt

1 12-ounce jar premade tomato sauce of your choice or sundried tomato and basil sauce, page 137

1. Bring a pot of water to a rapid boil and cook the shells until soft; drain and let cool.
2. Spray a small sauté pan, preferably nonstick, with olive oil and cook the onion and garlic about 3 minutes, until translucent and soft. Remove from the heat.
3. Meanwhile, in a medium mixing bowl, combine the ricotta cheese, chopped baby spinach, and half of the Parmesan cheese. Stir well to combine. Add the seasonings, onion, and garlic and combine well.
4. Brush a layer of tomato sauce on the bottom of a baking dish. Stuff each shell with an equal amount of filling and place in the baking dish. Cover the shells with the sauce and bake at 350 degrees for 15 minutes.
5. Sprinkle with remaining Parmesan cheese and continue baking for 5 minutes. Serve warm with extra sauce on the side.

Nutrition Facts:

Serving Size 2 shells, Calories 170, Fat 5g, Saturated Fat 4g, Cholesterol 23mg, Protein 16g, Carbohydrate 33g, Sugars 6g, Dietary Fiber 4g, Sodium 743mg

New Orleans Vegetarian Jambalaya

This dish is hard to find without meat, so that's the treat here—a healthy and vegetarian version of a typically meaty recipe.

YIELD: 8 SERVINGS

- 2 green bell peppers, diced
- 1 cup chopped celery
- 1 large onion, chopped
- 4 cloves garlic, chopped
- 28-ounce can tomatoes with juice
- 1 teaspoon salt
- 1 teaspoon pepper
- 1 teaspoon hot pepper sauce (red Tabasco)
- 1 teaspoon basil, dried
- 1½ cups frozen peas
- 2½ cups brown rice, cooked according to package directions
- 1½ cups white beans
- 2 cups cubed firm tofu
- 1 pinch red pepper flakes

1. In a large pot, simmer the peppers, celery, onion, garlic, tomatoes, salt, pepper, pepper sauce, basil, and peas for 15 minutes.
2. Place half of the vegetable mixture in a baking dish. Sprinkle in rice, add the remaining vegetable mix on top of the white beans, firm tofu, and stir to combine.
3. Cover and bake for 30 minutes at 350 degrees
4. Finish with the dried pepper flakes, sprinkled on top.

Nutrition Facts:

Serving Size 1½ cups, Calories 216, Fat 2g, Saturated Fat 0g, Cholesterol 0mg, Protein 12g, Carbohydrate 38g, Sugars 8g, Dietary Fiber 8g, Sodium 559mg

Vegetarian Stuffed Cabbage

Many who have tried this recipe prefer it to the more common meat-filled cabbage because it is not heavy to digest but still has the same texture and taste as if it were prepared with meat.

YIELD: 10 CABBAGE ROLLS

CABBAGE ROLLS

1 large head green cabbage

20 ounces of Garden Burgers (hamburger style), or packaged soy meat (can be found in produce section, a recommended brand is called Gimme Lean beef flavor)

1 medium onion, grated

1 medium carrot, grated

1 cup cooked brown rice

2 teaspoons tomato sauce

1 teaspoon honey or brown sugar

2 egg whites

1 garlic clove, minced

2 teaspoons minced parsley

1 teaspoon dried thyme

1 teaspoon pepper

SAUCE

2 cups thinly sliced cabbage leaves

1 onion, sliced thinly

1 garlic clove, minced

2 teaspoons canola oil

½ cup water or vegetable broth

1 28-ounce can crushed tomatoes in purée

¼ cup apple cider vinegar

¼ cup dark brown sugar or honey

1 whole clove

1 bay leaf

1. To prepare the cabbage rolls, bring a large pot of water to a boil. Core the cabbage and place it in the water. Cook until the leaves become translucent and can be removed from the head, about 5 to 7 minutes. Remove the cabbage from the water.

2. When cool enough to handle, carefully remove about 10 large leaves from the head. Reserve the rest of the cabbage.
3. In a large bowl, break up the Garden Burgers into small pieces. Add the remaining cabbage roll ingredients and mix thoroughly to form a solid mixture.
4. Assemble the rolls by placing each cabbage leaf stem- or vein-side down. Put about ½ cup of the soy mixture at the wide end of each cabbage leaf. Fold the sides over the filling toward the center and then roll the cabbage leaves up lengthwise. Place each roll in a large casserole or baking dish, seam-side down. Cover and set aside in the refrigerator.
5. To make the sauce, cut the reserved cabbage into thin slices. In a medium saucepan, sauté the cabbage, onion, and garlic in oil. Add the broth and tomatoes in purée and stir well. Bring to a boil. Turn the heat to a medium simmer and add the vinegar, sugar or honey, clove, and bay leaf and cook, covered, until the cabbage is soft and the sauce is fully cooked, about 20 to 30 minutes.
6. Pour the sauce over the cabbage rolls, cover tightly with a lid or foil and bake in the oven at 350 degrees for 25 to 30 minutes, until sauce is bubbly.

Nutrition Facts:

Serving Size 1 roll, *Calories* 179, *Fat* 1g, *Saturated Fat* 0g, *Cholesterol* 0mg, *Protein* 12g, *Carbohydrate* 12g, *Sugars* 16g, *Dietary Fiber* 6g, *Sodium* 597mg

Quick Tip

This recipe is actually easier to make than it looks. However, it can be thrown together even more quickly if you make the sauce ahead of time. This dish can also be made and frozen in servings. It will keep for at least a month in the freezer.

Gayle's Feel-Good Facts

When we eat food that is comforting we feel satisfied both physically and emotionally. Pasta dishes with cheese fall into the comfort-food category. Having them on hand in the freezer is a great way to take care of yourself when you come home late and don't want to cook. What a treat—no cooking and a hot healthy meal. Then all you need to do is unwind and relax.

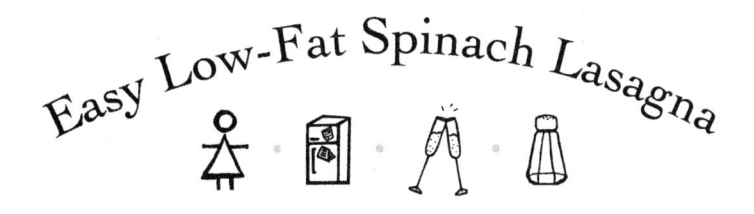

Easy Low-Fat Spinach Lasagna

Using precooked noodles and jarred sauce makes this recipe easy to make, and it is a perfect dish to freeze. If you have more time, feel free to pre-boil whole-wheat lasagna noodles.

YIELD: 6 SERVINGS

- 1 26-ounce jar prepared tomato sauce, your choice of flavor
- 8 ready to cook lasagna noodles or 4 ready to cook lasagna noodle squares (whether you use squares or noodles will depend on the brand you choose) or 8 fresh whole-wheat noodles
- 2 cloves fresh garlic, chopped fine and sautéed
- 1 pound fat-free ricotta
- 1 pound baby spinach, stemmed, washed, and dried
- 1 large red pepper, roasted and chopped
- 1 1/2 cups shredded nonfat or part-skim mozzarella
- 1 cup chopped basil
- 1/2 teaspoon Italian seasoning
- 1/4 cup (1 ounce/30 g.) freshly grated Parmesan cheese
- Ground pepper to taste

1. Generously cover the bottom of an 8 x 8-inch baking pan with tomato sauce. Lay noodles on top of sauce, covering the entire bottom of the pan. Coat the top of the noodles with sauce to cover.
2. In a small bowl mix the garlic and the ricotta cheese so they are well combined.
3. Spread a third of the ricotta cheese on top of the noodles.
4. Sprinkle one third of the spinach, one third of the red pepper, half of the mozzarella, 2 tablespoons of basil, a pinch of Italian seasoning, and 1 tablespoon of Parmesan cheese over the ricotta.
5. Put a second layer of noodles on top of the cheese and vegetables. If the noodles have grooves, lay the grooves going in the opposite direction of the first layer (this helps catch the sauce).
6. Cover the second layer of noodles generously with sauce. Make sure the noodles are well covered. Then repeat steps 3 and 4.
7. Continue this way for an additional layer. On top of the last layer of vegetables, sprinkle $1/4$ teaspoon ground pepper, then cover with noodles. Cover the noodles with the sauce, remaining mozzarella cheese, and Parmesan cheese.
8. Cover the pan with foil and bake at 350 degrees for 45 minutes. Remove the foil and bake for another 10 minutes, or until the top is lightly browned. Let cool 5 to 10 minutes before cutting.

Nutrition Facts:

Serving Size $1/6$ lasagna, Calories 398, Fat 11g, Saturated Fat 4g, Cholesterol 24mg, Protein 33g, Carbohydrate 47g, Sugars 5g, Dietary Fiber 11g, Sodium 1147mg

Gayle's Feel-Good Facts

Basil, a prevalent herb in Italian cooking, has health benefits aside from its fresh taste and fragrant smell. Basil contains flavonoids that act against cancer and an oil called estragole, which can inhibit growth of unwanted parasites and bacteria.

POULTRY

Gayle's Feel-Good Facts

Most people eat one vegetable or less with dinner and fill up on the protein and starch. A healthier alternative that will allow you to cut back on calories and boost the protective nutrients in your day is to serve your entrées with two vegetable sides (one can be a starter) and a grain or starch.

Almond Chicken
with Mustard-Thyme Sauce

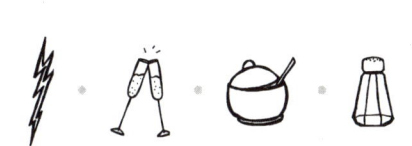

This is a simple, elegant recipe that is quick to make. Just make sure you have the seasoning and almonds on hand.

YIELD: 4 SERVINGS

CHICKEN

1 cup almonds, skinless

1 egg

4 boneless skinless chicken breast halves

SAUCE

1½ cups chicken broth

1½ tablespoons Dijon mustard

1 tablespoon chopped thyme or 1 teaspoon dried

¼ teaspoon granulated sugar

Pinch of salt

Pepper to taste

1. Place the almonds in a pie pan or cookie sheet and broil for 2 minutes until lightly browned and toasted. Watch the nuts to make sure they do not burn.
2. When the nuts are cool, chop them by hand with a knife or in a food processor into small pieces and place on a large plate.
3. In a small bowl, beat the egg. Dip each chicken breast in egg and then coat with the chopped almonds.
4. Spray or coat a large nonstick sauté pan with oil, heat over medium-high heat, and sauté the chicken breast, 5 minutes on each side. Place the breasts on a baking sheet and bake at 350 degrees for 15 minutes.
5. While the chicken is baking make the sauce. Combine the chicken broth with the mustard, thyme, and sugar. Cook uncovered over medium heat to reduce by a third. Season with salt and pepper. Keep warm until you are ready to serve.
6. Serve sauce over chicken.

Nutrition Facts:

Serving Size 1 chicken breast plus ¼ sauce, *Calories* 205, *Fat* 7g, *Saturated Fat* 1g, *Cholesterol* 72mg, *Protein* 27g, *Carbohydrate* 3g, *Sugars* 1g, *Dietary Fiber* 1g, *Sodium* 461mg

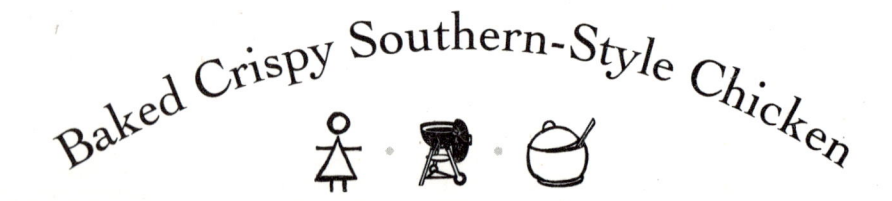

Baked Crispy Southern-Style Chicken

An old-time favorite made light—not exactly the same as deep fried, but close enough that you will enjoy every bite. Plus, you won't have to worry about unwanted, unhealthy fats.

YIELD: 6 SERVINGS

CHICKEN

¼ teaspoon paprika

1 garlic clove, minced

1 bay leaf, crumbled

2 tablespoons honey

½ teaspoon crushed dried thyme

¼ teaspoon cayenne

½ teaspoon kosher or table salt

2 cups nonfat yogurt, plain

3 whole skinless, boneless chicken breasts, halved

½ cup all-purpose flour

1 cup panko bread crumbs (available in Asian and gourmet supermarkets)

½ teaspoon dried parsley flakes

1 egg

½ teaspoon baking powder

¼ teaspoon baking soda

oil spray

HONEY MUSTARD DIPPING SAUCE

½ cup Grey Poupon mustard

½ cup clover honey

1. In a small bowl combine paprika, garlic, bay leaf, honey, thyme, cayenne, and salt. Add the yogurt to the spice mixture and mix well.
2. Coat the chicken with the yogurt mixture and lie flat in a baking dish. Refrigerate for 2 hours.
3. Combine flour, bread crumbs and dried parsley in a large shallow dish.
4. Beat the egg, baking powder, and baking soda in a large shallow bowl.
5. Shake off excess yogurt marinade from the chicken breast and drop in the flour mixture to coat, shaking off excess flour. Dip the chicken breast in the egg mixture, allowing excess egg to drip off, then coat pieces in flour again.
6. Place the chicken breast on a baking sheet that has been sprayed with canola oil or lightly coated with canola oil.
7. Spray the top of the chicken breast with oil.
8. Bake at 400 degrees for 35 to 40 minutes until done.
9. Serve with coleslaw (page 98) and Baked Potato Fries (page 204).

Nutrition Facts:

Serving Size 1 chicken breast, *Calories* 295, *Fat* 4g, *Saturated Fat* 1g, *Cholesterol* 52mg, *Protein* 13g, *Carbohydrate* 51g, *Sugars* 33g, *Dietary Fiber* 1g, *Sodium* 898mg

---

Gayle's Feel-Good Facts

In certain recipes, to maintain the integrity of the food, it is important to make an exception and use all-purpose flour or semolina flour pasta. In fried chicken, you can feel free to substitute whole-wheat flour; however, it will lend itself to a less "traditional" Southern-fried taste. As long as using refined flours is the exception and not the rule, it will not have a great impact on your health.

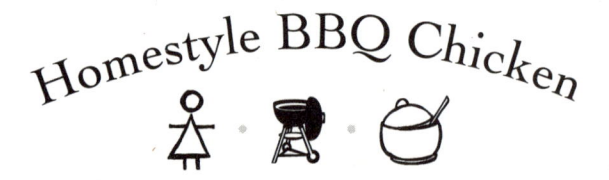

Homestyle BBQ Chicken

BBQs are always fun. This zesty sauce is sure to give any food a great flavor. You can also use it on salmon, shrimp, and meat.

YIELD: 4 SERVINGS

CHICKEN

1 3-pound chicken, cut into 8 pieces, skin and fat removed

¼ cup chicken broth

BBQ SAUCE

⅓ cup catsup

¼ cup hoisin sauce

1 tablespoon cider vinegar

1 tablespoon molasses

1 teaspoon reduced-sodium soy sauce

1 teaspoon honey

2 teaspoons pineapple juice

⅛ teaspoon cayenne or 2 dashes Tabasco

1. Arrange the chicken pieces in a baking dish with chicken broth and cover with foil. Heat in a 350 degree oven for 10 to 15 minutes, until the chicken is moist and partially cooked.
2. In a small bowl combine the sauce ingredients.
3. With tongs, remove the chicken from the baking dish and place on a baking sheet covered with foil. Using a brush, generously coat both sides of each piece of chicken with the BBQ sauce.
4. Grill over medium-high heat or broil, basting with BBQ sauce often, until the chicken is glazed on the outside and no longer pink inside, about 5 to 7 minutes on each side.
5. Serve warm or cold.

Nutrition Facts:

Serving Size 2 pieces of chicken, *Calories* 488, *Fat* 11g, *Saturated Fat* 3g, *Cholesterol* 239mg, *Protein* 74g, *Carbohydrate* 19g, *Sugars* 7g, *Dietary Fiber* 0g, *Sodium* 820mg

Gayle's Feel-Good Facts

The skin on poultry is where most of the unhealthy saturated fats can be found. With this recipe, you will impart flavor and not miss the skin. Dark-meat chicken has more fat than light meat, but without skin, both are good, low-fat choices.

Chicken Cacciatore

You can't go wrong serving this dish. It is easy and tastes good anytime, especially as a leftover.

YIELD: 4 SERVINGS

½ tablespoon olive oil

8 boneless, skinless chicken thighs (about 1 pound)

1 large onion, finely chopped

3 cloves garlic, minced

10 ounces sliced mushrooms

1 red pepper, cubed

1 green pepper, cubed

¼ cup white wine (optional)

8 ounces diced Italian plum tomatoes in juice

1 teaspoon Italian seasoning

½ teaspoon salt

¼ teaspoon black pepper

2 tablespoons chopped parsley

2 tablespoons chopped basil (optional)

¼ cup grated Parmesan cheese (optional)

4 cups brown rice or whole-wheat spaghetti, cooked

1. Heat the oil in a large skillet (preferably nonstick) on medium-high heat and brown the chicken quickly on all sides, 2 to 3 minutes. When finished, remove the chicken and place in a baking dish.
2. Reduce the heat to medium. Sear the onions and garlic for 2 minutes, then add the mushrooms and peppers. Sauté until the mushrooms and peppers are cooked and the onions are translucent and soft. Add the white wine and tomatoes with juice. Mix in the Italian seasoning, salt, and pepper.
3. Pour the sauce over the chicken. Cook at 350 degrees for 20 minutes, until the chicken is cooked through.
4. To serve, sprinkle with parsley, basil, and Parmesan cheese. This dish can be served over brown rice or whole-wheat spaghetti.

Nutrition Facts:

Serving size 2 chicken thighs plus sauce, *Calories* 555, *Fat* 17g, *Saturated Fat* 5g, *Cholesterol* 83mg, *Protein* 38g, *Carbohydrate* 60g, *Sugars* 7g, *Dietary Fiber* 5g, *Sodium* 603mg

Chicken Pot Pie

A low-fat twist on a high-fat favorite comfort meal. This meal can be frozen for up to three months.

YIELD: 6 SERVINGS

2 pounds skinless, boneless chicken breast

1 teaspoon canola oil

1 large onion, finely chopped

2 shallots, minced

1 leek, white part only, washed and cut into $1/4$-inch rounds

$3/4$ cup white wine

$1/2$ pound fresh mushrooms, quartered

4 medium carrots, cut into $1/2$-inch slices

1 cup chicken broth

1 teaspoon fresh thyme or $1/2$ teaspoon dried

1 teaspoon lemon peel

4 medium parsnips, peeled and cut into $1/2$-inch slices

1 large potato, cleaned, peeled and cut into $1/2$-inch cubes

1 cup green beans, cut into 1-inch pieces

1 cup fresh or frozen peas

3 tablespoons cornstarch mixed with 3 tablespoons water

1 teaspoon fresh parsley or $1/2$ teaspoon dried

1 teaspoon salt

1 teaspoon white pepper

12 sheets of phyllo dough

1. Trim the breasts of all fat and cut into 1-inch pieces. Set aside, covered, in the refrigerator.
2. Heat oil in a dutch oven or sauté pan over medium heat. Add the onion, shallots, and leek. Cook for a minute, then add the wine and cook vegetables until soft.
3. Add the mushrooms and carrots, stir, and cook for 5 minutes.
4. Add the broth, thyme, and lemon peel, and bring to a simmer.
5. Add the chicken, parsnips, and potato and simmer for half an hour, skimming broth from time to time.
6. Add the green beans and peas and cook for 5 minutes. Stir ¼ cup broth into the cornstarch mixture until smooth. Be sure to get rid of any lumps. Stir the cornstarch mixture into the pot. Simmer for 2 minutes, stirring constantly. Add parsley and salt and pepper. Remove from the heat.
7. Transfer the contents to individual baking dishes or one casserole dish.
8. Remove a leaf of phyllo from the roll of dough and place it on top of the pot pie mixture. Spray with olive oil or brush with olive oil lightly. Lay another leaf of dough over the first and spray with oil or brush lightly with oil. Repeat procedure until you have four layers. Lightly coat the top layer with oil. Trim the dough with a sharp knife so that it fits around the casserole dish.
9. If using individual casserole dishes, use a ½ sheet of dough for each casserole and layer ½ on top of each leaf until you have four layers, then trim off excess with a sharp knife.
10. Cook covered with aluminum foil for 20 minutes. Uncover the pot pie and continue to cook for an additional 10 minutes.

Nutrition Facts:

Serving Size 1 pie or ⅙ casserole, *Calories* 495, *Fat* 6g, *Saturated Fat* 1g, *Cholesterol* 88mg, *Protein* 44g, *Carbohydrate* 62g, *Sugars* 10g, *Dietary Fiber* 9g, *Sodium* 878mg

Chicken Roulade with Crumb-Nut Crust

This is an excellent party dish or special dinner dish, as it takes a bit of prep time. You can speed up the prep time with frozen and pre-sliced vegetables and preparing some of the filling ahead of time. If you prefer, this recipe can be made with turkey breast instead.

YIELD: 4 SERVINGS

- ¼ cup pistachio nuts
- 1 pound chopped frozen spinach leaves, thawed
- ½ teaspoon freshly grated nutmeg
- 2 cups sliced white mushrooms (if you desire, use pre-sliced mushrooms)
- ½ cup white wine
- ½ small sweet onion, sliced very thin
- 1 teaspoon thyme
- 1 teaspoon salt
- 1 teaspoon ground white pepper
- 4 boneless, skinless chicken breasts, about 6 ounces each, trimmed of fat
- 2 egg whites
- ¼ cup whole-wheat flour
- ¼ cup breadcrumbs

1. Grind the pistachios in the food processor or chop with a knife until finely ground. Set aside.
2. Steam the spinach or wilt it in a hot sauté pan. Chop finely, sprinkle with nutmeg, and set aside.
3. Heat a sauté pan, spray lightly with oil, and add the mushrooms. Sauté the mushrooms for 2 to 3 minutes and add ¼ cup of the white wine. Cook until well browned and most of the juice has evaporated. Put mushrooms into the processor and blend until mixture resembles a coarse paste. Set aside.

4. Spray the sauté pan again with oil and toss in sliced onions. Sear well, about 2 to 3 minutes, and add the remaining ¼ cup of white wine. Cover the pan and cook until the onion is soft and caramelized (browned). Set aside and allow to cool.

5. In a small bowl mix together the thyme, salt, and white pepper and set aside.

6. Place each chicken breast between 2 sheets of plastic wrap and pound with the flat side of a meat pounder from the center out so that the thickness is uniform, about a quarter inch. Be careful not to tear the meat.

7. Sprinkle some of the thyme mixture on each chicken breast. Place the breast vertically on a cutting board or flat surface. Place a quarter of the chopped spinach lengthwise on the bottom third of the breast.

8. Arrange a quarter of the mushroom mixture on top of the spinach, then a quarter of the onions.

9. Roll the roulades carefully, lengthwise, pushing in on the top after each turn to secure a tight roll. Each roulade should have about two or three turns. Wrap in plastic wrap and roll each tightly to secure the sides. Refrigerate for about 20 minutes.

10. Place the egg whites in a shallow bowl and the flour in a separate bowl.

11. Combine the plain breadcrumbs with pistachio nuts in a small bowl.

12. Unwrap the roulades from the plastic wrap, dredge in flour and shake off excess. Dip in egg white then in the pistachios to lightly cover on both sides.

13. Spray a roasting pan or baking sheet with oil spray. Place the roulades, folded side down, on the pan and bake at 350 degrees until firm, about 15 to 20 minutes.

14. To serve, slice the ends off each roulade, then slice each roulade on the bias into thirds. Arrange decoratively on a plate. Suggested side dishes are wild rice pilaf and roasted vegetables.

Nutrition Facts:

Serving Size 1 roulade, *Calories* 328, *Fat* 10g, *Saturated Fat* 2g, *Cholesterol* 90mg, *Protein* 26g, *Carbohydrate* 32g, *Sugars* 0g, *Dietary Fiber* 1g, *Sodium* 811mg

Duck Breast with Port Wine Sauce

Duck breast is often not low-fat; however, recently at some butchers and gourmet supermarkets you can find skinless duck breast. This can be a great treat if you are someone who loves duck but have stayed away from it due to its fat content.

YIELD: 4 SERVINGS

4 ½-pound skinless duck breasts, found frozen or at your butcher

½ teaspoon salt

¼ teaspoon black pepper

¼ teaspoon white pepper

4 allspice whole berries, crushed

½ teaspoon honey

½ teaspoon orange peel, grated

¼ teaspoon thyme

1 teaspoon olive oil

PORT WINE SAUCE

½ cup port wine

2 shallots, chopped fine

½ cup chicken broth

1. Trim the fat and skin from the duck breast.
2. Combine the salt, black and white peppers, allspice, honey, orange peel, thyme, and olive oil in a large bowl.
3. Add the duck breast to the seasoning and coat.
4. In a baking dish or large baking sheet that is coated with foil, bake the duck breast for 15 minutes, or until cooked through.
5. While the duck is cooking combine the port wine sauce ingredients in a saucepan and heat on medium heat. Pour the sauce over the duck before serving.
6. Serve with side dishes of choice, see page 199.

Nutrition Facts:

Serving Size 1 duck breast, *Calories* 382, *Fat* 7g, *Saturated Fat* 1g, *Cholesterol* 324mg, *Protein* 64g, *Carbohydrate* 5g, *Sugars* 4g, *Dietary Fiber* 0g, *Sodium* 555mg

Gayle's Feel-Good Facts

Duck breasts can be almost as lean as dark meat chicken. They make a nice change from chicken and have a hearty taste, so enjoy. But don't be deceived. Unless the duck breast is trimmed of skin and excess fat, it is not really considered low-fat. Beware if you are at a restaurant and think about ordering duck.

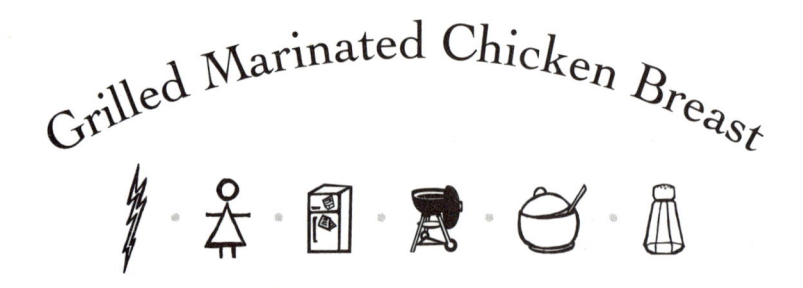

Grilled Marinated Chicken Breast

This simple marinade gives great flavor to the chicken without much effort You can serve it plain or put it in a salad. The marinade can also be used with fish. It is great with mashed potatoes and grilled vegetables.

YIELD: 4 SERVINGS

1 pound boneless, skinless chicken breasts

2 tablespoons lemon juice

2 cloves garlic, minced

¼ cup Dijon mustard

1 teaspoon finely chopped fresh rosemary or ½ teaspoon dried

1 teaspoon finely chopped fresh thyme or
½ teaspoon ground

1 teaspoon dried basil

1 teaspoon dried parsley

⅛ teaspoon salt

⅛ teaspoon pepper

½ cup chicken broth

1. Trim visible fat from the chicken. Mix the lemon juice, garlic, mustard, and herbs together in a medium mixing bowl. Rub over the chicken breasts and marinate for 2 hours in a baking dish or large bowl.
2. Grill on a hot grill, for about 5 minutes on each side, until the chicken is cooked through. Or, sauté in a nonstick skillet for 2 to 3 minutes on each side on medium-high heat to sear in flavor. Remove the chicken breast and heat on a baking sheet in a 350-degree oven for 6 minutes, until the chicken is cooked through.
3. Pour ½ cup of chicken broth into sauté pan to form a sauce with the chicken drippings. Pour the light sauce over the chicken and serve.

Nutrition Facts:

Serving Size 1 chicken breast, *Calories* 155, *Fat* 3g, *Saturated Fat* 0g, *Cholesterol* 66mg, *Protein* 28g, *Carbohydrate* 4g, *Sugars* 0g, *Dietary Fiber* 0g, *Sodium* 548mg

Quick Tip

When marinating fish, chicken, and meat, you can use a large Ziploc bag. This makes it easy to periodically shake the marinade so that it covers the food well and it also saves room in the refrigerator.

Roast Turkey with Sherry Cider Gravy

This is a low-fat, juicy way to make a turkey. Feel free to choose an organic bird, as they often have a better flavor than nonorganic.

YIELD: 12 SERVINGS

BASTING MIXTURE

¼ cup dry sherry

1 tablespoon olive oil

¼ cup apple cider

2 tablespoons apple butter

¼ teaspoon salt

½ tablespoon fresh chopped thyme

TURKEY

1 turkey cooking bag for up to 12 pounds

1 12-pound turkey with giblets

1 teaspoon kosher salt

1 teaspoon freshly ground black pepper

2 golden delicious apples, unpeeled, cored, and quartered

4 thyme sprigs

2 sage leaves

2 sprigs rosemary

1 medium onion, quartered

4 cloves of garlic

1¼ cups low-sodium chicken broth

2 cups apple cider

2 bay leaves

SHERRY CIDER GRAVY

2 tablespoons cornstarch

2 teaspoons Worcestershire

1 tablespoon minced parsley

Ground black pepper to taste

1. Position the oven rack in the lower third of the oven; preheat to 400 degrees. Cooking bags are meant to be used at 400 degrees, so you may want to put a thermometer in your oven to make sure it isn't running hot. Prepare a large roasting pan with a roasting rack.

2. In a small bowl mix together the basting mixture ingredients and set aside.
3. Remove the bag of giblets from the main and neck cavities of the bird and discard the liver and giblets. Rinse the turkey well and pat dry with a paper towel.
4. Rub the salt and pepper on the inside of the turkey. Then stuff the turkey with the apples, thyme sprigs, sage, rosemary, onions, and garlic.
5. Brush the outside of the turkey with the basting mixture, generously covering the bird. Reserve excess.
6. Place the turkey in the cooking bag breast side down. Place the turkey on the roasting rack. Close the bag loosely with the tie so that some steam can escape.
7. Coat the bottom of the pan with ¼ cup of the chicken broth and place the neck in the bottom of the pan. Let the bird roast for 30 minutes. Then, turn the bird over so the breast is facing up, lower the oven temperature to 325 degrees, and continue cooking for another 2 hours.
8. After 2½ hours of roasting, remove the turkey from the bag and pour the juice from the bag into the bottom of the roasting pan. Spray the roasting rack before putting the bird back on the rack to continue cooking for another hour. Baste the bird with the juices that are in the bottom of the pan. Add to the roasting pan the remaining 1 cup of chicken broth, ¼ cup of apple cider and the bay leaves.
9. Continue to baste the turkey with the remaining apple cider mixture every 30 minutes and continue roasting for another hour. The turkey is done when an instant-read thermometer registers 170 degrees when inserted into the thickest part of the thigh.
10. When the turkey is finished cooking, spill out the remaining juices from the cavity into roasting pan, discard neck, and set aside before removing the bird from the pan. Then place the bird on a carving board or serving platter and tent the turkey with foil to keep warm. Carve the turkey after it has rested for 20 minutes.
11. To make the gravy, skim off as much fat as possible from the juices that you reserved from the roasting pan using a large spoon, or if you have a gravy fat separator, you can use this tool.
12. In a small bowl, mix the cornstarch with some of the defatted drippings until well blended. Add this mixture and the Worcestershire to the roasting pan.

13. Bring the juices to a simmer over medium heat on the stovetop and keep stirring until it thickens. Add the parsley and pepper.
14. Pour into a gravy boat or small bowl; keep warm until ready to serve.

Nutrition Facts (with skin and including gravy):
Serving Size 1/12 of bird, Calories 441, Fat 14g, Saturated Fat 4g, Cholesterol 257mg, Protein 70g, Carbohydrate 5g, Sugars 3g, Dietary Fiber 0g, Sodium 329mg

Gayle's Feel-Good Facts

Cooking with wines and liquors is a good way to add flavor to foods, but keep in mind that only a small portion of the alcohol is burned off during cooking. Ask your doctor or pharmacist about having alcohol in food if you are on medication that should not mix with alcohol.

Sautéed Chicken Breast
with Wild Mushroom Sauce

This recipe is very popular with my cooking classes and tastes even richer the next day.

CHICKEN

4 5-ounces boneless, skinless chicken breasts, fat trimmed

3 tablespoons all-purpose flour

1/2 teaspoon freshly milled black pepper

2 tablespoons olive oil

WILD MUSHROOM SAUCE

2 cloves garlic, chopped fine

1 large portabella mushroom

6 ounces mixed mushrooms (cremini, porcini, shitake, buttom), sliced

2 tablespoons Madiera or red wine

1 cup chicken or vegetable broth

1 tablespoon chopped fresh thyme or 1 teaspoon dried

$1/2$ teaspoons chopped fresh rosemary or $1/2$ teaspoon dried

$1/2$ teaspoon salt

2 tablespoons chopped fresh Italian parsley

Pepper to taste

1. Place the chicken breast within a folded piece of plastic wrap; slightly flatten upper portion of each breast with the broad side of a chef's knife or hammer lightly with a kitchen mallet to flatten breasts so they cook more evenly.
2. On a piece of wax paper combine the flour and pepper. Lightly dredge each breast in seasoned flour (dredge just before cooking or flour coating will become gummy).
3. In a 12-inch skillet, heat oil over medium-low heat. Add the chicken and sauté until lighly golden, about 3 minutes on each side. Transfer the chicken to a serving platter and cover loosely with a tent of foil.
4. To make the sauce, spray the skillet with a light coating of oil and add the garlic. Turn the heat on low and cook until soft but not brown. Add the mushrooms and sauté over medium heat until tender, 3 to 5 minutes. Add the wine, broth, and seasonings. Simmer until the liquid is reduced by half (about 10 to 15 minutes).
5. Season with pepper to taste. Pour over chicken and serve.

Nutrition Facts:

Serving Size 15 oz chicken breast plus sauce, *Calories* 346, *Fat* 8g, *Saturated Fat* 1g, *Cholesterol* 82mg, *Protein* 32g, *Carbohydrate* 7g, *Sugars* 0g, *Dietary Fiber* 1g, *Sodium* 312mg

Traditional Turkey Meat Loaf

A low-fat version of a family favorite.

YIELD: 8 SERVINGS

2 slices whole-wheat bread	1 egg white
1 cup skim milk	1 carrot, peeled and finely ground
1 teaspoon canola oil	1 scallion, thinly sliced
1 small onion, finely diced	1 teaspoon salt
3 mushrooms, minced	1 teaspoon ground white pepper
1 clove garlic, minced	½ cup puréed canned tomatoes
2 tablespoons chopped parsley	1 tablespoon dark brown sugar
½ teaspoon dried thyme	1 tablespoon Dijon mustard
1½ pounds ground turkey (white meat)	1 tablespoon balsamic vinegar

1. Tear the bread into chunks and soak in the milk. Set aside.
2. Heat the oil in a nonstick skillet over medium heat. Add the onion, mushrooms, and garlic. Sauté until the vegetables are soft. Stir in the parsley and thyme.
3. In a large bowl, combine the ground turkey with the egg white, carrot, scallion, sautéed vegetables, salt, and pepper. Squeeze the excess milk from the bread and add the bread to the bowl. Mix with your fingers until just combined. Transfer the mixture to an 8 x 4-inch nonstick loaf pan and form into a smooth loaf.
4. In a small bowl, mix the tomatoes, brown sugar, mustard, and vinegar and put the mixture over the top of the loaf.
5. Bake for an hour at 375 degrees, or until the meat thermometer inserted into the center of the loaf registers 160 degrees. Let stand for 5 mintues before slicing.

Nutrition Facts:

Serving Size ⅛ *of meat loaf, Calories* 152, *Fat* 4g, *Saturated Fat* 2g, *Cholesterol* 62mg, *Protein* 17.5g, *Carbohydrate* 87g, *Sugars* 9g, *Dietary Fiber* 2g, *Sodium* 409mg (*without salt, Sodium* 142mg)

Bountiful Burger with Chipotle Catsup

The chipotle catsup gives this common burger a real Tex-Mex flavor boost. The burgers can be frozen and the catsup can keep in the refrigerator for up to a week. Chipotle peppers can be found in a can at the supermarket or gourmet store.

YIELD: 4 SERVINGS (4 BURGERS)

BURGER

½ red onion, finely chopped

1 pound ground turkey

½ teaspoon dried thyme

¼ cup chopped parsley

½ teaspoon salt

¼ teaspoon black pepper

¼ teaspoon Worcestershire

4 whole-wheat hamburger buns

4 slices of tomato

4 green leaf lettuce leaves

CHIPOTLE CATSUP (16 OZ)

1 cup diced onion

1 lb tomatoes, chopped

½ cup diced red pepper

1 whole chipotle pepper

1 teaspoon celery seeds

1 teaspoon mustard seeds

1 teaspoon cumin seeds

1 cinnamon stick

⅛ cup sugar

½ teaspoon paprika

¼ teaspoon allspice

½ teaspoon chili powder

¼ cup white vinegar

½ teaspoon salt

¼ teaspoon pepper, or more to taste

1. For the burgers, heat the oil in a medium skillet. When warm add the onions and sear until translucent, about 3 minutes.
2. Transfer the onion to a medium bowl. Add the ground turkey, thyme, parsley, salt, pepper, and Worcestershire and mix well.
3. Form 4 patties about ¾ inch thick. Either heat the grill or preheat the broiler and cook the patties, about 5 minutes on each side, or until cooked.
4. Add the buns to the grill or broil for the last minute of cooking, facedown, to warm.
5. Serve on a bun with lettuce, tomato, and chipotle catsup.
6. In a large pot, mix the onion, tomatoes, red pepper, and chipotle pepper. Simmer for 20 minutes, then purée and put back in the pot and simmer for 1 hour.
7. Place the seeds and cinnamon stick in cheesecloth and tie with twine. Add to the pot and simmer 20 minutes more.
8. Remove the cheesecloth and add the remaining ingredients to the pot. Simmer 45 minutes.
9. Add salt and pepper to taste.

Nutrition Facts:

Serving Size 1 burger plus 2 tablespoons catsup, *Calories* 398, *Fat* 13g, *Saturated Fat* 3g, *Cholesterol* 42mg, *Protein* 29g, *Carbohydrate* 42g, *Sugars* 5g, *Dietary Fiber* 2g, *Sodium* 665mg

Gayle's Feel-Good Facts

When shopping for lean meats, look for the round or loin cut of beef, pork, veal, and lamb. Other lean meats include some game: venison, rabbit, buffalo, and ostrich. Always trim visible fat from the meat, since it is the visible fat that is saturated, the fat that is most likely to raise your cholesterol. It is wise not to eat meat daily but one to two times a week, to limit saturated fats.

RED MEAT

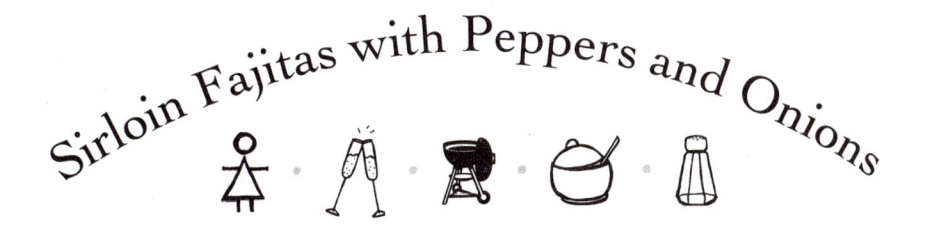

Sirloin Fajitas with Peppers and Onions

Fun for everyone to eat, this is a good way to use beef, as sirloin is lean and cooks quickly.

YIELD: 4 SERVINGS

MARINADE

½ teaspoon kosher salt

¼ teaspoon freshly ground black pepper

½ cup cilantro, chopped

2 tablespoons lime juice

½ teaspoon lime peel, chopped

3 garlic cloves, minced

1 teaspoon cumin

⅛ teaspoon cayenne

1 teaspoon olive oil

FAJITAS

1¼ pounds flank steak, well trimmed, sliced into ¼-inch thick strips

1 small onion, thinly sliced

1 red bell pepper, thinly sliced

1 green bell pepper, thinly sliced

4 large whole-wheat tortillas

½ avocado, sliced in eighths

1 cup low-fat tomato salsa

½ cup non-fat or low-fat sour cream

1. Combine the marinade ingredients in a medium bowl and stir to combine.
2. Mix the steak with half the marinade and place in the refrigerator for at least 1 hour.
3. In a large skillet coated with cooking spray, sauté the onion and peppers on medium heat until soft, about 6 minutes. While the vegetable mixture is cook-

ing, add 1 tablespoon of reserved marinade to the skillet. Stir the vegetables to mix with the marinade. Store the cooked vegetables in foil to keep warm.
4. Warm the tortillas according to the package directions
5. Spray the skillet again and warm on medium heat. Add the meat and cook on medium-high heat for 5 minutes. Place the steak in a large bowl to keep warm.
6. To serve, place equal portions of beef and pepper mixture in the center of a tortilla, divide up slices of avocado and distribute evenly to all servings, place 1 teaspoon of fat-free sour cream on top of meat, and roll up.
7. Serve with tomato and tomatillo salsa on the side.

Nutrition Facts:

Serving Size 1 fajita, *Calories* 233, *Fat* 8g, *Saturated Fat* 1g, *Cholesterol* 0mg, *Protein* 10g, *Carbohydrate* 32g, *Sugars* 9g, *Dietary Fiber* 12g, *Sodium* 638mg

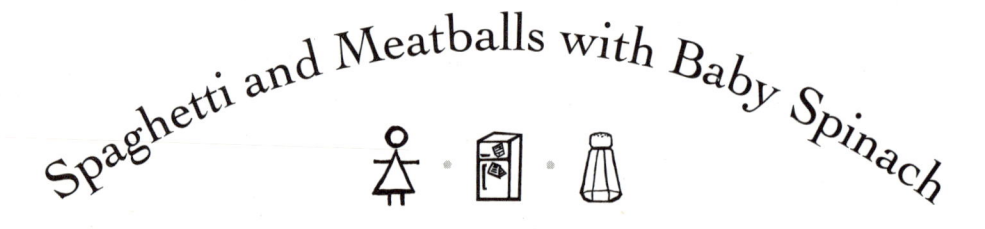

Spaghetti and Meatballs with Baby Spinach

Healthy and tasty, this low-fat translation of a family favorite is worth the time it takes to make. Plus you can premake and freeze the sauce and the meatballs, if you wish.

YIELD: 10 SERVINGS

MEATBALLS

½ cup (1 ounce) grated Parmesan cheese

1 cup unseasoned bread crumbs

½ cup skim milk

1½ cup low-sodium beef broth

½ cup chopped parsley

4 egg whites, beaten

2 teaspoons Italian seasoning

¼ teaspoon salt

¾ teaspoon crushed red pepper flakes

2 cloves garlic, minced

2 pounds ground round, extra lean

PASTA

1 pound cooked whole-wheat pasta

6 cups Sundried Tomato and Basil Sauce (page 137) or your favorite brand of jarred sauce

½ cup chopped basil

2 pounds baby spinach

1 cup grated Parmesan cheese (optional)

1. Mix together the Parmesan, bread crumbs, milk, ½ cup of the beef broth, parsley, egg whites, Italian seasoning, salt, pepper flakes, and garlic in a large mixing bowl.
2. Add the ground round. Stir well to combine with the bread crumb mixture.
3. Shape the mixture into about 32 meatballs (2 inches in diameter). You can use two spoons to scoop out the meat mixture or a 2-ounce scoop.
4. Coat a baking sheet with nonstick cooking spray. Place the meatballs on the baking sheet so they are not touching one another.
5. Cover the bottom of the pan with the remaining cup of beef broth (you may not need all of it). Bake at 400 degrees for 20 minutes, or until the meatballs are just cooked through.
6. In a large skillet heat the Sundried Tomato Sauce on medium heat. When warm, add the basil and spinach. Place the meatballs in the sauce to keep warm. Add the cooked spaghetti and serve hot with a sprinkle of Parmesan cheese if desired.

Nutrition Facts:

Serving Size 4 *meatballs plus* 2 *ounces pasta, Calories* 574, *Fat* 19g, *Saturated Fat* 7g, *Cholesterol* 64mg, *Protein* 91g, *Carbohydrate* 64g, *Sugars* 4g, *Dietary Fiber* 11g, *Sodium* 1551mg *(To reduce sodium—omit salt and use low-sodium tomato sauce and bread crumbs without salt. This will reduce the sodium to ~500mg/serving.)*

Veal Marsala

Quick and elegant, this is a dish your friends and family will rave over, and if you buy the precut mushrooms, it reduces your time on the prep.

YIELD: 4 SERVINGS

- 1 tablespoon plus 2 teaspoons olive oil
- 2 tablespoons finely chopped shallots
- 1 tablespoon minced fresh garlic
- 1 (8-ounce) package mushrooms, thinly sliced, or pre-sliced mushrooms
- 6 tablespoons vegetable broth
- 4 5-ounce veal medallion halves or veal prepared for scallopine
- 1 teaspoon salt, divided
- 1 teaspoon black pepper, divided
- ½ cup all-purpose flour
- ½ cup Marsala wine
- 2 tablespoons low-fat evaporated skim milk
- ½ teaspoon chopped fresh thyme or ¼ teaspoon dried
- 1 tablespoon chopped Italian parsley

1. Heat a large nonstick skillet with 2 teaspoons of the olive oil over medium-high heat; add the shallots and garlic, sauté for 1 minute, then add mushrooms. Sauté for 1 minute.
2. Add 3 tablespoons of the vegetable broth to the skillet and cook for 4 minutes, until the mushroom are slightly browned and the moisture evaporates. Remove the mushroom mixture from the pan and set aside.
3. If the veal is not flattened when purchased, place each veal medallion between 2 sheets of heavy-duty plastic wrap. Pound to a ¼-inch thickness using a meat mallet or rolling pin. Sprinkle both sides of the veal with ¼ teaspoon salt and ¼ teaspoon pepper.
4. Place the flour in a shallow dish and dredge veal halves in flour. Set aside.
5. Heat the remaining tablespoon of oil in the skillet over medium-high heat. Add the veal; cook 1 minute on each side, or until lightly browned. Remove the veal from pan.

6. Return the mushroom mixture to the pan and add the rest of the vegetable broth and wine, scraping the pan to loosen browned bits.
7. Bring the mixture to a boil, reduce heat, and simmer for 2 minutes, or until reduced by ¼. Stir in the evaporated low-fat milk, thyme, and parsley.
8. Return the veal to the pan and cook until thoroughly heated, 1 to 2 minutes. Serve veal and sauce with Wild and Brown Rice Pilaf (recipe page 214) or whole-wheat pasta.

Nutrition Facts:

Serving Size 1 veal medallion, *Calories* 352, *Fat* 11g, *Saturated Fat* 2g, *Cholesterol* 228mg, *Protein* 34g, *Carbohydrate* 21g, *Sugars* 5g, *Dietary Fiber* 2g, *Sodium* 840mg

Gayle's Feel-Good Facts

Meat meals are generally slightly higher than 30% fat per serving. But, when you put the meal with the side dishes, the entire meal will be less than 30% fat.

Moroccan Lamb Stew

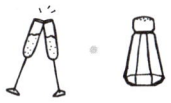

I enjoy making this dish for family gatherings or family-style dinner parties.

YIELD: 12 SERVINGS

1 tablespoon olive oil

2 cloves garlic, thinly sliced

1 large onion, diced

1 large carrot, diced

1 teaspoon cinnamon

½ teaspoon ground cumin

½ teaspoon ground thyme

4 pounds lamb shoulder, trimmed of all fat, cubed into 2-inch chunks

½ cup dry red wine

1 cup beef broth

1 cup slivered almonds

½ pound pitted prunes

¼ pound dried apricots

3 tablespoons honey

½ teaspoon salt

½ teaspoon black pepper

12 cups of Wild and Brown Rice Pilaf (page 214)

1. In a large soup or broth pot heat the oil and sauté the garlic, onion, carrots, cinnamon, cumin, and thyme. Cook until the garlic and onions are soft, about 2 to 3 minutes. Add the meat and stir to combine with the seasoning mixture.
2. Add the wine and broth, and bring to a boil over high heat, then reduce the heat and gently simmer, partially covered, over medium-low heat for 30 minutes.
3. Stir in the almonds, prunes, apricots, and honey.
4. Cook until the lamb is tender, about 30 minutes longer. Serve warm with brown rice.
5. Season with salt and pepper.

Nutrition Facts:

Serving Size 5 ounces lamb plus sauce and 1 cup rice, *Calories* 602, *Fat* 17g, *Saturated Fat* 4g, *Cholesterol* 97mg, *Protein* 39g, *Carbohydrate* 73g, *Sugars* 19g, *Dietary Fiber* 7g, *Sodium* 215mg

Rack of Lamb with Herbs and Garlic

Lamb is always tasty. This quick recipe can be served for company or a special dinner. The seasoning of the bread crumbs really dresses up this dish.

YIELD: 4 SERVINGS

1 French-cut lean rack of lamb loin chops or baby rack of lamb loin chops (about 1½ pounds, an 8-rib rack), trimmed of all visible fat

¼ teaspoon salt

⅛ teaspoon pepper

⅓ cup Grey Poupon mustard

1 tablespoon olive oil

2 garlic cloves, minced

1 shallot, minced

2½ teaspoons herbs de Provence

½ cup bread crumbs

Rosemary sprigs (optional)

1. Trim fat from the lamb. Season the lamb with salt and pepper.
2. Mix the mustard, oil, garlic, shallot, and ½ teaspoon of the herbs de Provence in a small bowl until well combined.
3. Place the lamb on a foil-lined baking sheet, rounded side up. Spread the mustard mixture evenly over the lamb. Refrigerate uncovered. (For best results, marinate the lamb for at least 6 hours.)
4. Mix the bread crumbs with the remaining 2 teaspoons of herbs de Provence and the olive oil. Press the bread crumbs on the outside of the lamb. Insert a meat thermometer into the thickest part of the lamb.
5. Bake at 450 degrees for 30 to 45 minutes, or until desired degree of doneness is reached. (Medium-rare is 145 degrees, medium is 160 degrees, and well-done is 170-180 degrees.)
6. Garnish with rosemary sprigs if desired.

Nutrition Facts:

Serving Size 2 chops, *Calories* 306, *Fat* 10g, *Saturated Fat* 4g, *Cholesterol* 112mg, *Protein* 37g, *Carbohydrate* 7g, *Sugars* 0g, *Dietary Fiber* 0g, *Sodium* 820mg

Gayle's Feel-Good Facts

Herbs de Provence, a blend of thyme, savory, rosemary, and marjoram, is used widely in southern France. It is an excellent blend to use with meat because it adds a robust flavor that combines well with the meat. Plus the balance of herbs eliminates the problem of having one herb overpower the others. Although it is a combination of stronger flavor herbs, herbs de Provence can be used on salmon and chicken as a light seasoning.

PORK

Pork Loin Stuffed with Dried Fruit

Pork loin is almost as lean as chicken breast and makes a great alternative when you are looking to add variety to your low-fat repertoire.

YIELD: 6 SERVINGS

- 1 cup mixed dried fruit (apples, pears, apricots, cherries)
- 1 teaspoon ground sage
- 1½ teaspoons chopped thyme
- ½ cup brandy
- 1 boneless pork loin (2 pounds), butterflied by butcher
- ½ teaspoon salt
- 1 teaspoon white pepper
- 2 teaspoons olive oil
- 2 shallots, chopped
- ⅔ cup red wine
- 1 teaspoon Dijon mustard

1. Coarsely chop the dried fruit and add the sage and ½ teaspoon of the thyme. In a small bowl mix the dried fruit mixture with the brandy. Let sit for 20 to 30 minutes. Drain the fruit from the brandy and reserve the brandy. Save the brandy.
2. Open the pork loin so it is almost lying flat. Spread the marinated fruit in the center of the pork loin. Roll and fold the stuffed pork loin so it is reshaped into a tight cylinder. Tie the meat in even sections by wrapping butcher's twine around the roast and making a secure knot. Cut the twine and tie a second knot 1 inch away from the first. Repeat. Repeat the tying process on the roast until you have 5 to 6 ties securing the filling and holding the roast in shape.
3. Sprinkle the roast with salt and pepper on all sides and rub with 1 teaspoon of olive oil.
4. Roast at 450 degrees for 10 minutes on a rack in a roasting pan. Lower heat to 350 and cook 1 hour more.
5. While the pork loin is cooking, in a small sauté pan, sauté shallots in the remaining teaspoon of olive oil, add the reserved brandy and wine, and simmer until reduced by half. Add the mustard. Slice the pork loin and serve with the sauce.

Nutrition Facts:

Serving Size 1 pork loin with sauce, *Calories* 318, *Fat* 10g, *Saturated Fat* 3g, *Cholesterol* 89mg, *Protein* 33g, *Carbohydrate* 7g, *Sugars* 0g, *Dietary Fiber* 1g, *Sodium* 297mg

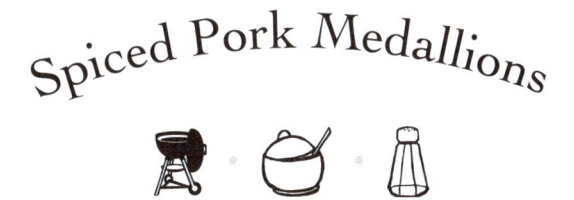

Spiced Pork Medallions
with Cranberry-Orange Sauce

The robust meaty flavors of pork work well with sweeter, fruity sauces. This is an easy recipe that tastes as though you spent hours preparing it.

YIELD: 4 SERVINGS

SPICE RUB

1 teaspoon dark brown sugar

1 teaspoon dried savory

1 teaspoon salt

½ teaspoon ground cinnamon

½ teaspoon ground white pepper

⅛ teaspoon ground cloves

½ teaspoon onion powder

½ teaspoon dried thyme

¼ teaspoon nutmeg

CRANBERRY-ORANGE SAUCE

1 tablespoon minced shallot

¼ cup white wine

1 cup chicken broth, defatted

1½ cups orange juice

1-pound bag fresh or frozen and thawed cranberries

1 cinnamon stick

Zest of one orange (about 1 tablespoon)

MARINADE

4 5-ounce pork loin medallions, visible fat removed

Juice of 1 lemon (about 1 tablespoon)

2 teaspoons minced garlic

2 teaspoons minced ginger

1 tablespoon honey

1. In a small bowl, mix together all the ingredients for the spice rub and set aside. To make cranberry-orange sauce, spray a medium sauce pan with oil and sear shallot for 2 minutes. Add wine, reduce by ½. Add chicken broth, orange juice, cranberries, and cinnamon stick and simmer until berries burst. Remove from heat, remove cinnamon stick and add more juice or broth if sauce is too thick. Season with orange zest. Set aside.
2. Make shallow diagonal slashes in pork loins, about 1 inch apart along the grain of the meat. Place the meat in a shallow baking dish. In a small bowl, combine 1 tablespoon of spice rub, lemon juice, garlic, ginger and honey. Rub over meat, on both sides. Marinate covered at room temperature for 15 minutes, or up to 4 hours, depending on the time you have.
3. Spray grill rack with oil or heat broiler. Place pork on grill or broiler and cook 5 minutes on each side, or until pork is cooked through.
4. Serve with Cranberry-Orange Sauce on top of each breast.

Nutrition Facts:

Serving Size 1 pork loin plus sauce, *Calories* 408, *Fat* 12g, *Saturated Fat* 5g, *Cholesterol* 101mg, *Protein* 36g, *Carbohydrate* 33g, *Sugars* 24g, *Dietary Fiber* 6g, *Sodium* 692mg

FISH AND SEAFOOD

Asian Marinated Tuna Loin

YIELD: 4 SERVINGS

MARINADE

1 cup lite teriyaki sauce

¼ cup dry sherry

2 tablespoons minced ginger

1 clove garlic, minced

Juice of 1 lime

Juice of 1 lemon

¼ cup chopped scallions, whites only

1 tablespoon honey

¼ teaspoon cayenne

4 5-ounce tuna loin steaks (yellowfin, albacore, or bigeye)

WASABI SAUCE

2 tablespoons rice wine vinegar

2 tablespoons sherry wine vinegar

⅓ cup mirin

2 tablespoons low-sodium soy sauce

1 tablespoon sesame oil

1 tablespoon light brown sugar

1 tablespoon minced ginger

1 teaspoon minced garlic

2 tablespoons chopped cilantro

1 to 2 tablespoons wasabi paste or powder

1. To make marinade: Combine the teriyaki, sherry, ginger, garlic, lime and lemon juices, scallions, honey, and cayenne. In a large shallow bowl, marinate the tuna for at least 3 hours.
2. To make wasabi sauce: Combine the wine vinegars, mirin, soy sauce, sesame oil, and brown sugar. Mix until the sugar dissolves. Stir in the ginger, garlic, and cilantro. Add the wasabi at the last minute.
3. Grill the tuna on a well-oiled grill on all sides, or sear in hot nonstick skillet on high on all sides, for 1 to 2 minutes so that the tuna remains medium-rare to medium. After the tuna is cooked, spoon a little sauce over it and serve remaining sauce as a dipping sauce on the side.

Nutrition Facts:

Serving Size 1 tuna loin with marinade and sauce, *Calories* 316, *Fat* 5g, *Saturated Fat* 0g, *Cholesterol* 83mg, *Protein* 47g, *Carbohydrate* 14g, *Sugars* 3g, *Dietary Fiber* 0g, *Sodium* 263mg

Gayle's Feel-Good Facts

Knowing what fish to eat these days can be confusing, because of all the press around mercury and pollutants in fish. Fish is healthy to eat because it contains omega-3 fats, which aid in reducing the risk of heart disease and cancer. It is recommended that you eat three to five servings of fish a week, but it is important to avoid fish that are high in mercury.

I have limited the fish recipes in this book to those fish that are considered safe to eat. Below is a list of fish that the FDA has deemed high in mercury content along with the recommendation for eating them. If you are pregnant or breast-feeding do not eat the fish in the avoid list and limit those in the high-mercury category. Pregnant and breast-feeding women should not exceed .2 ppm of mercury a day.

AVOID (EAT NO MORE THAN ONCE A MONTH):
CONTAIN > .7 PPM OF MERCURY
Tilefish
Swordfish
Shark
King mackerel

HIGH IN MERCURY (EAT NO MORE THAN ONCE A WEEK):
CONTAIN .4 TO .7 PPM OF MERCURY
Blue fish
Lobster (northern United States)
Marlin
Orange roughy
Red snapper
Saltwater bass
Trout, freshwater
Tuna (fresh or canned white albacore)

MODERATE IN MERCURY (EAT NO MORE THAN TWICE A WEEK):
CONTAIN .2 TO < .3 PPM OF MERCURY
Grouper
Halibut
Sablefish
Sea trout

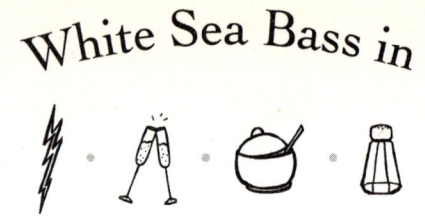

White Sea Bass in Tomato Basil Shallot Sauce

This mild fish blends well with the basil and tomato sauce and is quick to prepare.

YIELD: 4 SERVINGS

4 4-ounce sea bass filets

4 teaspoons olive oil

1 teaspoon salt

1 teaspoon pepper

4 cups chopped tomatoes

4 cups canned tomato purée without added salt

4 tablespoons minced fresh basil

4 teaspoons minced shallots (about 4 shallots)

1. Coat each filet in oil and sprinkle each with ¼ teaspoon of the salt and pepper.
2. In a large bowl mix together chopped tomatoes, tomato purée, and 3 tablespoons of the fresh basil and shallots.
3. Place the fish in a large skillet or baking dish. Pour the sauce over the fish. Bake at 375 degrees for 4 minutes, or until fish flakes easily when tested with a fork.
4. Sprinkle the remaining tablespoon of basil and shallots over the fish and serve hot.

Nutrition Facts:

Serving Size 1 filet with sauce, *Calories* 323, *Fat* 8g, *Saturated Fat* 1g, *Cholesterol* 60mg, *Protein* 33g, *Carbohydrate* 33g, *Sugars* 21g, *Dietary Fiber* 8g, *Sodium* 1367mg

Crab Cakes

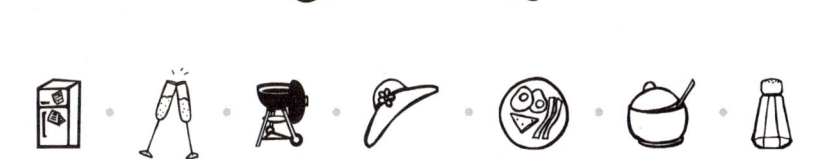

This recipe can be a main meal or prepared smaller for party hors d'oeuvres. The taste and the amount of crabmeat make these a real crowd pleaser.

YIELD: 6 THREE-OUNCE CRAB CAKES OR 18 ONE-OUNCE CRAB CAKES

1 pound fresh lump crabmeat (Dungeness, blue, or king)

2 egg whites

1 small red bell pepper, finely diced

½ cup corn kernels

¼ cup chopped flat leaf parsley

2 scallions, chopped

2 tablespoons fat-free mayonnaise

1 teaspoon Old Bay seasoning

1 teaspoon Worcestershire

1 teaspoon Dijon mustard

1 teaspoon fresh lemon juice

2 dashes Tabasco

1 cup panko (Japanese bread crumbs) or fresh bread crumbs

1. Preheat the oven to 375 degrees.
2. Pick over the crabmeat to remove any bits of shell or cartilage. Do not shred the crabmeat; leave in meaty chunks.
3. Beat the egg whites to soft peaks. Set aside.
4. In a mixing bowl, gently combine the crabmeat, pepper, corn, parsley, scallions, mayonnaise, Old Bay, Worcestershire, mustard, lemon juice, and Tabasco. Fold in the egg white mixture and ¼ to ½ cup of the panko.
5. Divide the mixture into 6 portions and form into rounded patties. The patties should just sick together and be somewhat delicate.
6. Roll each patty lightly in the remaining panko, flatten slightly into a cake, and place on a parchment-lined or nonstick baking sheet. Bake for 12 minutes, or until lightly puffed and browned.

Nutrition Facts:

Serving Size 1 3-ounce crab cake, *Calories* 146, *Fat* 2g, *Saturated Fat* 1g, *Cholesterol* 113mg, *Protein* 16.5g, *Carbohydrate* 15g, *Sugar* 2g, *Dietary Fiber* 1g, *Sodium* 500mg

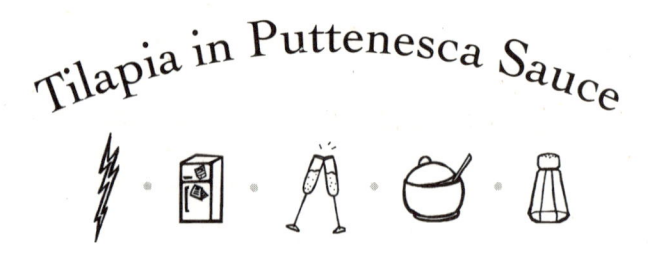

Tilapia in Puttenesca Sauce

Tilapia is a tender white fish that is low in mercury. This is a Mediterranean sauce packed with pungent olives and capers that impart an excellent flavor when combined with tomato. Once you learn how to make this sauce, you can also use it with chicken.

YIELD: 4 SERVINGS

1 tablespoon olive oil

¼ cup chopped onions

2 cloves garlic, chopped

¼ cup red wine, optional

2 tablespoons vegetable broth

¼ cup chopped kalamata olives

1 tablespoon capers

2 cups peeled canned tomatoes, diced

1 tablespoon fresh thyme or 1 teaspoon dried thyme

2 tablespoons chopped basil

¼ teaspoon salt

Ground pepper to taste

4 5-ounce tilapia steaks

1. In a large nonstick, oven-safe skillet, heat the oil on medium until warmed, about 2 to 3 minutes. Once heated, cook the onions and garlic for 1 to 2 minutes, until tender.
2. Add the wine and broth to slow the cooking of the garlic. Cook until the liquid is reduced by half.

3. Add the olives, capers, tomatoes, thyme, basil, salt, and pepper to the sauté pan and stir well.
4. Place the tilapia steaks into the sauté pan. Spoon the sauce over the tilapia.
5. Wrap the handle of the skillet with foil and place the sauté pan in the oven at 350 degree. Cook the fish until it flakes, approximately 12 to 15 minutes.
6. Serve with Wild and Brown Rice Pilaf (page 214) and your choice of vegetables.

Nutrition Facts:

Serving Size 1 filet of fish with sauce, *Calories* 443, *Fat* 12g, *Saturated Fat* 2g, *Cholesterol* 91mg, *Protein* 36g, *Carbohydrate* 6g, *Sugars* 1g, *Dietary Fiber* 1g, *Sodium* 508mg

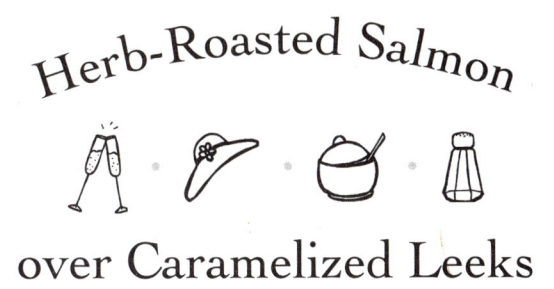

Herb-Roasted Salmon over Caramelized Leeks

This recipe sounds fancy, but it is really easy. Just take it one step at a time.

YIELD: 4 SERVINGS

4 5-ounce salmon filets, (Alaskan wild)

1 teaspoon salt

1 teaspoon ground black pepper

2 teaspoons of olive oil

1 teaspoon Grey Poupon mustard

1 tablespoon dried thyme

1 teaspoon tarragon

½ teaspoon white pepper

1 tablespoon chopped parsley

2 leeks, julienned

½ cup white wine

1. Sprinkle salmon filets with salt and pepper. Combine 1 teaspoon of the oil and the mustard, brush over the tops of the salmon filet.
2. Mix together the thyme, tarragon, white pepper, and parsley. Generously coat the top of each filet with 1 tablespoon of the mixed herb mixture.
3. Spray a large nonstick skillet with oil. Place salmon in skillet skin side or bottom side down. Cook in oven for 15 minutes at 350 degrees, until fish is cooked through.
4. Heat nonstick skillet, spray with 2 teaspoons of oil, add leeks. Stir quickly. Mix well, stir, and then add wine. Cover skillet and let leeks simmer until wine has evaporated and leeks are soft and slightly caramelized. About 8 to 10 minutes.
5. Place salmon filet over leeks to serve. You can serve either roasted vegetables and yukon gold mashed potatoes or wild rice pilaf as side dishes.

Nutrition Facts:

Serving Size 1 filet, *Calories* 312, *Fat* 13g, *Saturated Fat* 2g, *Cholesterol* 73mg, *Protein* 36g, *Carbohydrate* 6g, *Sugars* 1g, *Dietary Fiber* 1g, *Sodium* 658mg

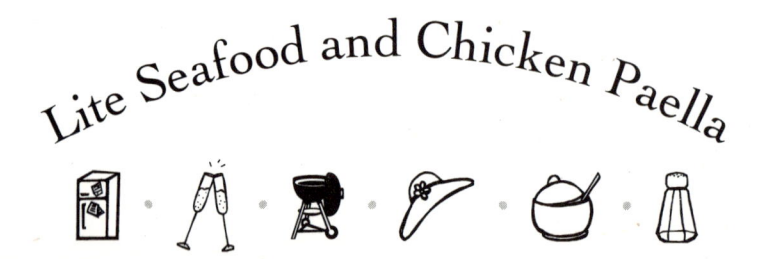

Lite Seafood and Chicken Paella

To make this a vegetarian recipe, just omit all the chicken and seafood and add 2 pounds of firm tofu. Also, feel free to add 2 cups of cooked garbanzo or white beans.

YIELD: 8 SERVINGS

1 pound boneless, skinless chicken breasts

1 teaspoon paprika

1 pound large shrimp (about 16), deveined, with tails removed

16 large sea scallops

1½ pounds monkfish

2 teaspoons mild chili powder

3 tablespoons canola oil

2 medium onions, diced

2 roasted red peppers, diced

1 jalapeno pepper, seeded and minced

2 cloves garlic, minced

1 28-ounce can chopped, seeded tomato and their juice

½ teaspoon chopped oregano

½ teaspoon chopped thyme

2 bay leaves

1 teaspoon sugar

½ teaspoon salt

6 tablespoons chopped cilantro

5 cups chicken or vegetable broth

½ teaspoon saffron threads

3 cups Arborio rice

¼ cup white wine

2 cups frozen green peas

2 medium scallions, minced

1. Sprinkle the chicken pieces with the paprika. Broil or grill until just cooked, about 8 minutes. When the chicken has cooled, cut each breast on the bias into thin slices and set aside.
2. Season the shrimp, scallops, and monkfish with the chili powder. Cover with plastic wrap and refrigerate.
3. Heat 2 teaspoons of the oil in a medium saucepan. Add the onions, red pepper, jalapeno pepper, and garlic and sauté. Add the tomatoes, oregano, thyme, bay leaves, sugar, and salt. Simmer, uncovered, until most of the liquid evaporates. Stir in 2 tablespoons of the cilantro. Set aside.
4. In a small saucepan bring the broth to a boil, add the saffron, and simmer over low heat. Add the tomato mixture and white wine, and stir. Reserve to be used in the next step.
5. In a large skillet, heat the remaining 1 teaspoon of oil, add the rice, and stir constantly until the rice is slightly toasted, or opaque, about 1 to 2 minutes. Slowly add the broth to the rice, 1 cup at a time, stirring constantly until the

liquid is almost absorbed. This will take about 15 to 20 minutes. When the rice is cooked it will be tender and plump. Add the peas and scallions. Season to taste with salt. Remove the pan from the heat.

6. Arrange the chicken, scallops, monkfish, and shrimp over the rice mixture. Cover with foil and bake for 7 minutes. Sprinkle with the scallions and remaining cilantro and serve.

Nutrition Facts:

Serving Size 1½ cups *Calories* 543, *Fat* 9g, *Saturated Fat* 2g, *Cholesterol* 185mg, *Protein* 58g, *Carbohydrate* 53g, *Sugar* 7g, *Dietary Fiber* 5g, *Sodium* 694mg (*without salt, sodium* 560mg)

Quick Tip

To shorten this paella recipe, you can purchase saffron or paella rice in a box at your market along with the sofrito base. Sofrito base can be found in a jar in the Spanish section of your supermarket. Sofrito is an authentic Spanish sauce that is made by sautéing tomatoes, green peppers, onions, and garlic in olive oil. Then, creating this delicious dish is simply a matter of cooking the seafood and chicken and mixing peas, scallions, chopped tomato, rice, and seasoning.

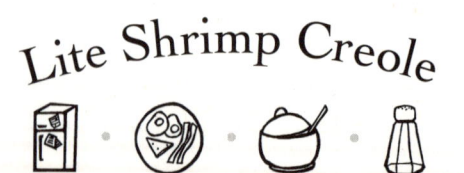

Lite Shrimp Creole

This recipe is sure to warm you up on a cold day. It can also be kept frozen for up to three months.

YIELD: 5 CUPS

SEASONING MIX

1 tablespoon paprika

2 teaspoons dried basil

1½ teaspoons onion powder

1½ teaspoons garlic powder

1 teaspoon salt

1 teaspoon dried mustard

½ teaspoon pepper

½ teaspoon oregano

½ teaspoon thyme

¼ teaspoon white pepper

⅛ teaspoon cayenne

1½ cups chopped onion

1 cup chopped green pepper

2 teaspoons olive oil or oil spray

½ cup chopped celery

3 bay leaves

1½ cups apple juice

1 teaspoon minced garlic

2 cups peeled diced tomatoes

½ cup tomato sauce

1 cup vegetable broth

1 pound medium shrimp, cleaned and deveined

1. Combine all the ingredients for the seasoning mix. Season the shrimp with 2 teaspoons of the mix and set aside.
2. Preheat the skillet and add olive oil or spray skillet with oil. Add the onions, peppers, celery, bay leaves, and 3 tablespoons of the seasoning mix.
3. Stir and cook until the vegetables start to brown. Add 1 cup of the apple juice and the garlic to deglaze the pan. Cook until the liquid evaporates.
4. Add the tomatoes and remaining seasoning mix and cook 2 minutes. Stir in the tomato sauce, broth, and remaining ½ cup of apple juice. Scrape the skillet and bring to a boil. Cook for 7 to 8 minutes.
5. Add the shrimp and cook until just pink, about 4 minutes. Serve over Wild and Brown Rice Pilaf (page 214).

Nutrition Facts:

Serving Size 1 cup, *Calories* 186, *Fat* 5g, *Saturated Fat* 0g, *Cholesterol* 140mg, *Protein* 26g, *Carbohydrate* 82g, *Sugars* 11g, *Dietary Fiber* 4g, *Sodium* 1011mg

Potato-Crusted Halibut with White Wine Sauce

When you put a crust on fish, it helps retain the fish's moisture, keeping it tender and succulent. Potatoes make an excellent crust because their flavor does not overpower the flavor of the fish.

YIELD: 4 SERVINGS

FISH	SAUCE
4 5-ounce halibut filets	1 tablespoon olive oil
1 teaspoon salt	¼ cup minced shallots
1 teaspoon white pepper	½ cup white wine
2 Yukon gold potatoes, peeled	½ cup vegetable broth
4 teaspoons olive oil	½ cup diced tomatoes
	2 tablespoons minced tarragon or 1½ teaspoons dried
	1 tablespoon chopped parsley

1. Season fish with salt and pepper.
2. Using a mandolin or food processor, coarsely shred the potatoes immediately before cooking. Spread the potatoes on a paper towel and press to get them as dry as possible. Divide the potatoes into 4 equal piles.
3. A nonstick skillet is very helpful for this dish. Each fish will be cooked individually in the pan. To cook each fish, oil the pan with 1 teaspoon of olive oil and heat the pan on medium heat. When the pan is hot, spread half of one pile of potatoes in the pan in a circle and cook for 2 to 3 minutes. Lay a filet on the

potatoes top down. Cook for several minutes until the potatoes firm up. Use a large spatula to lift the fish out of the pan and place in a baking dish so the bottom side is down. Repeat with the remaining 3 fish.

4. Sprinke the fish with more white pepper and place in a 350-degree oven and cook for 10 minutes, until the fish is cooked through.
5. While the fish is cooking, in a sauté pan, heat ½ teaspoon olive oil and sauté the shallots for 1 minute. Add the wine and cook until the wine is reduced by half. Add the vegetable broth, diced tomatoes, and tarragon. Reduce the sauce by half. Stir in remaining olive oil.
6. Pour the sauce over the fish on each plate to serve. Garnish with fresh tarragon and parsley leaves if desired.

Nutrition Facts:

Serving Size 1 filet, Calories 313, Fat 10g, Saturated Fat 1g, Cholesterol 41mg, Protein 29g, Carbohydrate 19g, Sugars 2g, Dietary Fiber 1g, Sodium 783mg

Salmon with Creamy Lime Dressing

An easy, quick, and tasty dinner that will taste like you slaved for hours. The yogurt makes an excellent coating for the fish. You can also try the lime dressing on chicken breast.

YIELD: 4 SERVINGS

LIME DRESSING

¼ cup honey

1 cup nonfat plain yogurt

¼ cup fresh lime juice

1 tablespoon minced ginger

1 tablespoon minced garlic

1 tablespoon minced mint

SALMON

4 5-ounce salmon steaks or filets (preferably Pacific or Alaskan)

16 green grapes, sliced in half

1. Combine the honey, yogurt, lime juice, ginger, garlic, and mint in a glass bowl and whisk until creamy. Set half of the dressing aside to serve with the cooked salmon.
2. Coat the salmon steaks or filets with the remaining dressing and refrigerate for 1 to 2 hours.
3. Preheat the oven to 375 degrees or prepare the grill for cooking.
4. Cook the salmon for 15 to 20 minutes (20 minutes per inch of salmon, 10 minutes each side).
5. Warm the excess creamy lime dressing in a small pan on low while the salmon is cooking (3 to 5 minutes).
6. Sprinkle the sliced green grapes on top of the salmon and serve with extra dressing on the side.

Nutrition Facts:

Serving Size 1 filet, Calories 349, Fat 13g, Saturated Fat 1g, Cholesterol 99mg, Carbohydrate 38g, Sugars 24g, Dietary Fiber 0g, Sodium 55mg

Gayle's Feel-Good Facts

It was recently reported that farm-raised salmon contains a greater amount of PCBs (polycholorinated biphenyls), cancer causing chemicals from the environment. When tested it was found the European farm-raised fish had higher levels of PCBs than American farm-raised fish, though both had higher levels of PCBs than wild salmon. To reduce your exposure to PCBs, when buying farm-raised salmon, look for the country of origin on the label, or better yet, purchase wild.

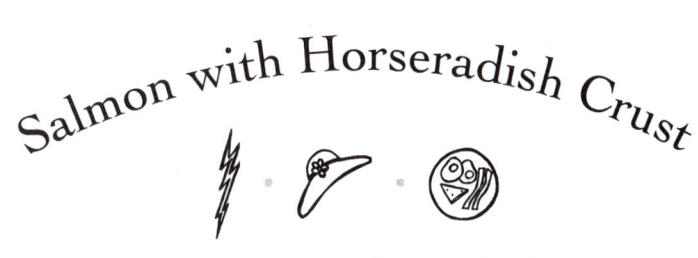

Salmon with Horseradish Crust
on Arugula Salad

Quick and elegant, this dish is packed with flavor, and will impress both family and friends.

YIELD: 4 SERVINGS

- 1 cup panko (Asian bread crumbs) or fresh bread crumbs
- 2 teaspoons nonfat yogurt
- 3 teaspoons canola oil
- 2 teaspoons chopped flat leaf parsley
- ½ cup prepared white horseradish or ¼ cup grated fresh horseradish

- 4 6-ounce salmon filets (use wild if possible)
- 1 tablespoon Dijon mustard
- 1 shallot, minced
- 1 clove garlic, minced
- 4 seeded and diced fresh plum tomatoes with their juice

4 tablespoons balsamic vinegar

½ teaspoon salt

½ teaspoon fresh ground black pepper

½ teaspoon sugar

4 cups cleaned and stemmed coarsely chopped arugula

1. Mix the fresh bread crumbs with the yogurt, 1 teaspoon of the canola oil, parsley, and horseradish. If the mixture is too dry, add more horseradish or yogurt. Set aside.
2. Brush the top of each salmon filet with Dijon Mustard and place in a baking dish.
3. Spread the horseradish mixture on top of each filet.
4. Place the filets in the oven and bake at 350 degrees for 5 to 8 minutes, or until the topping is golden brown.
5. Heat a sauté pan with the remaining 2 teaspoons of canola oil and sauté the shallots and garlic. Cook for 1 minute then add the tomatoes and vinegar and stir. Season with salt, pepper, and sugar. Add the arugula and cook until just wilted.
6. Divide the arugula mixture into 4 portions and arrange in the center of each plate.
7. Place a long spatula just under the skin of the salmon filet and remove from the baking dish. The salmon should lift off easily from its skin.
8. Place the salmon on top of the arugula salad. Serve hot.

Nutrition Facts:

Serving Size 1 filet with sauce, *Calories* 369, *Fat* 13g, *Saturated Fat* 2g, *Cholesterol* 94mg, *Protein* 38g, *Carbohydrate* 21g, *Sugars* 4g, *Dietary Fiber* 2g, *Sodium* 764mg

Gayle's Feel-Good Facts

The shredded root of horseradish is used as a homeopathic remedy to stimulate appetite and digestion.

Spicy Curry Grilled Scallops
with Mango Mint Salsa

Light and easy, this recipe is sure to please with its blend of sweet and spicy flavors.

YIELD: 4 SERVINGS

1½ teaspoon curry powder

1 teaspoon minced garlic

½ teaspoon minced thyme

1 teaspoon olive oil

1½ pounds large farmed sea scallops

½ teaspoon salt

SALSA

2 tablespoons fresh lemon juice

2 tablespoons fresh orange juice

2 medium mangoes, chopped

¼ cup sliced red radishes

2 jalapeno chilis, chopped with seeds

2 tablespoons chopped fresh mint

Black pepper to taste

1. Combine the curry powder, garlic, thyme, and oil and rub over the scallops in a large bowl.
2. To make the salsa, in a small bowl, combine the lemon and orange juice.
3. In a medium bowl, mix together the mangoes, radishes, and chilis. Pour the juice mixture over the mango mixture and combine well. Sprinkle with mint and black pepper.
4. Heat a nonstick skillet or skillet sprayed with oil spray until it is well warmed on high heat, about 2 to 3 minutes. Add the scallops and reduce heat to medium-high. Cook the scallops until they are firm to the touch, about 4 minutes. Season with salt and pepper. Serve hot with the salsa.

Nutrition Facts:

Serving Size 5 ounces, Calories 240, Fat 3g, Saturated Fat 0g, Cholesterol 56mg, Protein 29g, Carbohydrate 25g, Sugars 17g, Dietary Fiber 3g, Sodium 573mg

Trout with Pecan-Cornmeal Crust

Crunchy and light, the cornmeal crust adds a lovely Southern flair to this easy-to-use recipe. I recommend that you serve it with Sauteéd Greens with Garlic (page 220).

YIELD: 4 SERVINGS

CRUST

¾ cup cornmeal

1 tablespoon minced parsley

1 shallot, minced

¼ cup chopped pecans

1 tablespoon minced thyme or 1 teaspoon dried

¾ cup low-fat buttermilk

½ teaspoon salt

½ teaspoon black pepper

4 6-ounce rainbow trout filets

1. Blend together in a food processor or blender the cornmeal, parsley, shallot, pecans, and thyme until a blended meal forms. Do not overblend or the meal may get sticky. Place on a large plate when finished.
2. In a large bowl, mix together the buttermilk, salt, and pepper.

3. Dip each trout filet into the buttermilk and then into the cornmeal mixture. Place the trout on a nonstick or oil-sprayed baking sheet. Sprinkle extra cornmeal on top of the trout. Lightly spray the top of the trout with oil spray.
4. Bake at 400 degrees for 10 minutes, or until the fish flakes easily when tested with a fork. Serve with lime wedges.

Nutrition Facts:

Serving Size 1 trout, *Calories* 364, *Fat* 12g, *Saturated Fat* 3g, *Cholesterol* 86mg, *Protein* 34g, *Carbohydrate* 25g, *Sugars* 3g, *Dietary Fiber* 3g, *Sodium* 393mg

Gayle's Feel-Good Facts

Thyme, while a familiar and widely used herb, also has medicinal properties as an antiseptic, cough remedy, and digestive aid. In ancient times, thyme was used as a meat preservative.

8

Sides

Scrumptious sides are always a welcome accompaniment to a tasty entrée. Listed in this section are grain, starch, and vegetable sides. If you are looking to watch your weight, fill up on vegetables. There are charts to help you learn how to prepare tasty vegetables anytime by roasting, grilling, or steaming. I always recommend that you have two or more vegetables at a meal. This can include the starter as well.

Roasting or Grilling Individual Vegetables

Roasting brings out the sweetness of the vegetables and is one of the more tasty ways to enjoy cooked vegetables. Even people who don't like eating vegetables often find them much more enjoyable roasted or grilled. Whether you are roasting or grilling vegetables, you can use the same method. The chart below lists the vegetables that taste the best grilled or roasted, how to prepare them to be cooked, and how long to cook them.

To cook, place the sliced vegetables in a single layer on a nonstick or foil-lined baking sheet. If grilling, you can use foil or a grill pan to prevent the vegetables from falling into the grill. Before placing the vegetables on the pan or grill, spray with oil spray. If you choose to roast in the oven, heat the oven to 425 degrees. Your vegetables are roasted or grilled when they are soft and slightly browned. You can turn them when they are cooked halfway.

Quick Tip

While roasting imparts its own delicious flavor, you can add flavor to vegetables by tossing them in marinades before cooking. You can buy a marinade at the grocery store or try making your own by adding 2 teaspoons of fresh thyme or rosemary, or 1 teaspoon of herbs de Provence to balsamic vinegar.

VEGETABLE	PRREPARATION	COOKING TIMES
Grape tomatoes	Rinse and place whole on baking sheet	10 minutes
Beets	Scrub beats and trim ends, leave unpeeled	1 hour whole
	If roasting whole, mini, or full-size, peel when cooked	
	Sliced with skin	20 minutes
Miniature beets	unskinned	20 to 30 minutes
Red onions	Peel and cut into $1/4$-inch slices	20 minutes
Turnips	Peel, trim, and cut into $1/8$-inch slices	25 minutes
Carrots	Slice $1/4$-inch slices	20 minutes
Asparagus	Trim tough ends	20 minutes

Steaming Vegetables

Steaming vegetables is another good technique for cooking vegetables. When vegetables are very fresh, they can taste their best steamed without any sauce. Vegetables can be steamed in a metal steamer in a saucepan, an Asian bamboo steamer in a wok, or to speed them up, you can use a Japanese rice cooker, which is like a Crockpot.

VEGETABLE	PREPARATION	COOKING TIMES
Asparagus	Slice off rough ends before cooking; best if standing in an asparagus steamer; if not, use a large pot and a metal steamer so the asparagus can lie flat	Cook uncovered 5 minutes, then covered 7 to 10 minutes
Beans, green	Wash and snap ends off	15 to 20 minutes, until tender
Beets, small	Scrub the skin; do not peel	20 to 30 minutes, until tender but still firm
Broccoli	Cut off the rough bottom stalk or peel before cooking; cut into smaller florets.	10 to 20 minutes
Brussels sprouts	Wash well; cut off stems	12 to 15 minutes
Carrots	Scrub thoroughly or peel; cut off the ends; chop the carrots into bite-size pieces	12 to 15 minutes
Cauliflower	Core; remove the outer leaves; cut into florets	12 to 15 minutes

(continued)

VEGETABLE	PREPARATION	COOKING TIMES
Eggplant	Peel and slice; salt the slices to remove bitterness; let stand for 15 minutes, then rinse well	Steam for 3 to 5 minutes; if you are steaming eggplant in prep for grilling or roasting, steam for 3 minutes, then place in oven or on the grill
Fennel	Wash well, slice out core bulb	20 to 30 minutes
Greens	Wash well; remove bad leaves and stem if desired	5 to 8 minutes or until wilted; baby greens take half the time
Jicama	Peel the outside skin and cut off the brown stem; slice into equal-size pieces	8 to 15 minutes, or until tender but crisp
Mushrooms	Wipe with a damp towel or clean with a mushroom brush; cut off the ends	3 to 8 minutes
Okra	Wash; remove "fuzz" with a towel; remove the tips	3 to 8 minutes
Parsnips	Scrub well or peel; leave them whole or chop them into equal-size pieces	Whole: 20 to 40 minutes Cut: 5 to 15 minutes
Summer squash	Wash and trim each end; slice the squash horizontally or vertically into $1/4$-inch dice	5 to 10 minutes
Corn	Remove the husk; wash	Covered for 6 to 10 minutes

GRAIN AND STARCH SIDES

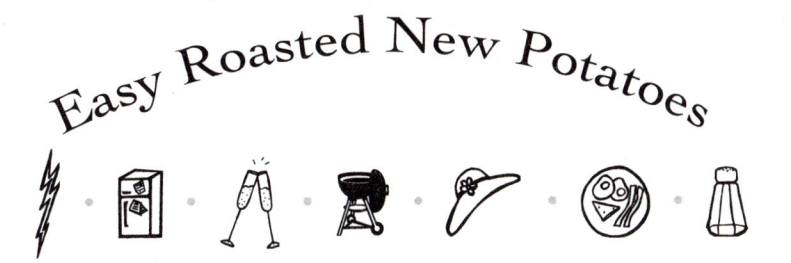

Easy Roasted New Potatoes

A simple and flavorful way to prepare potatoes for lunch, dinner, or a side at breakfast.

YIELD: 4 SERVINGS

1 pound new potatoes

1 tablespoon olive oil

2 cloves garlic, minced

3 tablespoons chopped assorted herbs (thyme, parsley, rosemary)

1 teaspoon salt

Black pepper to taste

1. Preheat the oven to 400 degrees.
2. Line a shallow roasting dish or pan with foil.
3. Cut the potatoes into quarters or halves. In a medium mixing bowl, coat the potatoes with oil, garlic, herbs, salt, and pepper.
4. Roast until slightly browned, about 25 minutes. Serve warm.

Nutrition Facts:

Serving Size ¼ pound, about ½ cup, Calories 137, Fat 1g, Saturated Fat 0g, Cholesterol 0mg, Protein 2g, Carbohydrate 24g, Sugars 0g, Dietary Fiber 2g, Sodium 539mg

Baked Potato Fries

Here you can choose your type of potato. I recommend either a Russet or sweet potato. The method for cooking the potatoes was adapted from a recipe I read in *Cooks* magazine.

YIELD: 6 SERVINGS

3 medium potatoes (about 8 ounces each), peeled and cut lengthwise into even-sized French fry strips

2 tablespoons canola oil

½ teaspoon salt

Ground black pepper to taste

oil spray

1. Arrange the oven rack on the lowest possible position. Preheat the oven to 475 degrees.
2. Place the potatoes in a large bowl and cover with hot tap water. Allow the potatoes to soak for 10 minutes.
3. Coat a heavy baking sheet with the oil and sprinkle salt and pepper over the baking sheet.
4. Drain the potatoes and pat dry thoroughly with a paper towel. Arrange the potatoes in a single layer on the baking sheet and spray the tops of the potatoes with oil spray. Cover the potatoes tightly with foil and bake for 5 minutes. Remove the foil and continue to bake until the potatoes are browned on the bottom, about 20 minutes. When the potatoes are cooked on one side, loosen with a spatula and flip them. Continue baking until the fries are crisp, about 5 to 10 minutes.
5. Season with salt and pepper. Serve hot.

Nutrition Facts:

Serving Size ½ cup, Calories 123, Fat 3g, Saturated Fat 0g, Cholesterol 0mg, Protein 2g, Carbohydrate 87g, Sugars 1g, Dietary Fiber 2g, Sodium 153mg

Gayle's Feel-Good Facts

White potatoes, long thought to have no nutritional value, are actually packed with vitamin C and potassium and are low in calories. Sweet potatoes, though not related to the white potato, are also loaded with potassium and vitamin C, as well as the protective nutrients vitamin E and betacarotene.

If you are on a low-carb diet, you will be happy to know that if you eat potatoes with the skin, the fiber from the skin limits the elevation of blood sugar caused by the potatoes. For those watching their carbs, you can feel comfortable eating one serving of potatoes, the equivalent of half a potato, along with your protein (meat, chicken, fish, or seafood). By combining food groups and the fiber from the potato skin, the impact on your sugar levels is greatly reduced.

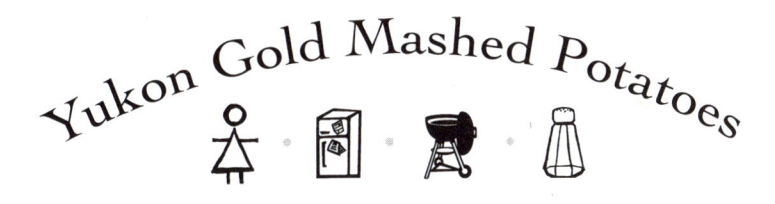

Yukon Gold Mashed Potatoes

YIELD: 6 SERVINGS

4 medium Yukon gold potatoes, peeled and cut into large cubes

1 cup evaporated skim milk

1 teaspoon salt

3/4 teaspoon white pepper

1. Place the potatoes in a saucepan and cover with cold water. Bring the water to a boil and cook the potatoes until soft, about 30 minutes.

2. Just before the potatoes are finished cooking, heat the milk in a small saucepan on low heat until warmed.
3. Run the potatoes through a food mill or blend until smooth in a food processor. In a large mixing bowl, mix the potatoes with the warm milk, salt, and pepper and serve.

Nutrition Facts:

Serving Size ⅓ cup, Calories 180, Fat 0g, Saturated Fat 0g, Cholesterol 1mg, Protein 6g, Carbohydrate 39g, Sugars 7g, Dietary Fiber 3g, Sodium 765mg

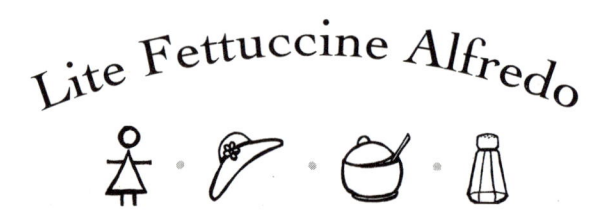

Lite Fettuccine Alfredo

I created this recipe for the Food Network as a challenge to come up with a low-fat version of a typically high-fat dish. It tastes just as rich as if it had cream in it. So enjoy indulging without the guilt!

YIELD: 12 SERVINGS

1 cup fat-free ricotta

1½ cups freshly grated imported Parmesan cheese

2½ cups skim milk

¼ cup arrowroot or cornstarch

1 teaspoon olive oil

6 quarts water

12-ounces fettuccine

1½ cups fat-free Parmesan cheese

Pinch of freshly grated nutmeg

1 teaspoon salt

Freshly ground black pepper to taste

2 tablespoons chopped Italian parsley

1. Blend the ricotta with the imported Parmesan cheese and mix well.
2. In a saucepan, whisk the milk and cornstarch or arrowroot. Heat over medium-high heat, stirring, until the mixture thickens and comes to a boil, about 10 minutes.
3. Bring 6 quarts of water to a boil. Add the olive oil and fettuccine. Cook until al dente.
4. Transfer the mixture to a medium metal bowl or to the top half of a double boiler and whisk in the ricotta mixture and fat-free Parmesan cheese. Season with nutmeg and salt. Add the freshly ground pepper to taste.
5. Drain fettuccine and toss with the sauce.
6. Serve hot. Garnish with parsley. Sprinkle chopped parsley on top of fettuccine and serve hot. Add more pepper and nutmeg if desired.

Nutrition Facts:

Serving Size ½ cup, Calories 205, Fat 4g, Saturated Fat 3g, Cholesterol 15mg, Protein 18g, Carbohydrate 23g, Sugars 5g, Dietary Fiber 0g, Sodium 725mg

Moroccan Spiced Couscous

Almost a meal, this couscous is packed with flavor and substance from the beans. Great for a party or BBQ as a side, this recipe makes quite a large portion. Feel free to freeze some. It will keep well for at least a month.

YIELD: 6 CUPS

2 teaspoons canola oil

2 medium zucchini, cubed

½ cup scallions, thinly sliced

2 teaspoons curry powder

2 teaspoons ground cinnamon

1 teaspoon cumin

½ teaspoon turmeric

¼ cup dry white wine

10 ounces Italian plum tomatoes, drained and finely chopped

2 cups cooked chickpeas

2 cups dried currants

1 teaspoon sugar

1 teaspoon salt

2 cups vegetable broth or water

1 6-ounce box whole-wheat couscous

1 cup frozen peas, thawed

1 cup chopped parsley

Juice and zest of 1 orange

1. Over a medium flame, heat the canola oil in a large deep skillet. Add the zucchini and scallions and cook for 2 minutes. Stir in the curry, cinnamon, cumin, and turmeric and cook for 30 seconds, stirring well to prevent burning.
2. Add the wine and cook until the liquid is reduced by half. Stir in the tomatoes, chickpeas, currants, sugar, and salt.
3. Add the broth and bring to a boil.
4. Remove the skillet from the heat, stir in the couscous, cover, and let stand for 5 minutes, or until the couscous has absorbed the liquid.
5. Gently fluff the couscous with a fork and fold in the peas and parsley. Add the juice and zest and mix well. Serve hot, cold, or room temperature.

Nutrition Facts:

Serving Size 1 cup, Calories 357, Fat 3g, Saturated Fat 0g, Cholesterol 0mg, Protein 12g, Carbohydrate 51g, Sugars 37g, Dietary Fiber 14g, Sodium 311mg

Gayle's Feel-Good Facts

Couscous is made of flour that has been precooked and dried, so it cooks quickly. Whole-wheat couscous contributes more fiber to your diet than the more common semolina-flour couscous.

Low-Fat Festive Stuffing

For those who prefer a stuffing instead of potatoes, here is a low-fat version that is sure to please your palate.

YIELD: 10 TO 12 SERVINGS

- 2 cups chopped onions
- 2 cups chopped celery
- 1/2 cup dry white wine
- 3 cups sliced button mushrooms
- 1/4 cup brandy or cognac, optional
- 2 Granny Smith apples, peeled and cubed
- 3/4 cup toasted chopped walnuts, optional
- 6 cups stale whole-grain bread cut into cubes
- 1 teaspoon salt
- 1 teaspoon pepper
- 1 teaspoon dried thyme
- 1 teaspoon freshly ground nutmeg
- 1/2 teaspoon dried sage
- 1/2 cup chopped Italian or flat leaf parsley
- 1/2 cup fat-free chicken or vegetable broth
- 1 egg white

1. Preheat the oven to 325 degrees.
2. In a large, deep skillet that has been warmed on medium heat, sauté the onions and celery for 30 seconds, then add the white wine and cook until the wine has evaporated and the vegetables are softened.
3. Transfer the vegetables to a large bowl. In the same skillet add the mushrooms and sauté on high heat. Add the brandy or cognac. Cook until the brandy has evaporated and the mushrooms exude their juices and are browned.
4. Add the mushrooms to the vegetables in the bowl, along with any liquid. Add the chopped apples, nuts, and bread cubes and toss lightly.
5. Sprinkle with salt and pepper, dried herbs, and chopped parsley.

6. Add the chicken or vegetable broth and egg white and toss again until blended. The mixture should be slightly moist but not mushy.
7. Place the stuffing into an ovenproof casserole dish and bake for 30 to 40 minutes, covered or use to stuff a turkey or other poultry.

Nutrition Facts:

Serving Size ½ cup, Calories 165, Fat 5g, Saturated Fat 1g, Cholesterol 0mg, Protein 5g, Carbohydrate 22g, Sugars 6g, Dietary Fiber 4g, Sodium 474mg

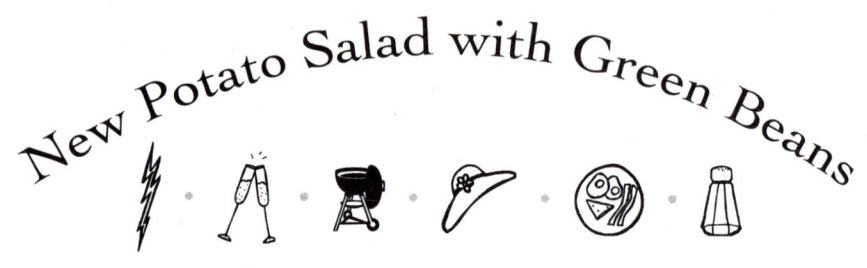

New Potato Salad with Green Beans and Toasted Pine Nuts

Potato salad is always a popular side, winter or spring. It can be served warm or cold. The nuts and green beans add a nice, fresh, nutty crunch to complete the mellow flavor of the potato.

YIELD: 8 SERVINGS

1 cup fresh green beans

32 ounces new potatoes, peeled and sliced ¼-inch thick (32 potatoes)

½ shallot, minced

¼ cup pine nuts, toasted

¼ cup rice wine vinegar

¼ teaspoon salt

¼ teaspoon black pepper

1 tablespoon Dijon mustard

2 tablespoons vegetable broth

1 tablespoon olive oil

¼ cup chopped parsley

2 tablespoons finley chopped scallions, whites only

1 tablespoon chopped dill

1. Cut the green beans into 1-inch pieces.
2. Place the potatoes in a large pot and cover with water. Bring to a boil, reduce to a simmer, and cook until tender but not falling apart, about 8 minutes. When the potatoes have cooked about 4 minutes, add the green beans to the water. Once cooked, drain and rinse the potatoes and green beans and let cool in a large mixing bowl.
3. For dressing, sauté the shallot in a small skillet that has been sprayed or lightly coated in oil until tender, about 2 minutes. Add the pine nuts to the pan and sauté the pine nuts for an additional 2 minutes. Place the cooked shallots and pine nuts in a small mixing bowl.
4. Add to the small mixing bowl the vinegar, salt, pepper, mustard, broth, and oil. Mix with a whisk until well blended.
5. Once the potatoes are cooled add the parsley, scallions, and dill. Mix well, then add the dressing.

Nutrition Facts:

Serving Size ½ *cup, Calories* 121, *Fat* 4g, *Saturated Fat* 0g, *Cholesterol* 0mg, *Protein* 4g, *Carbohydrate* 17g, *Sugars* 2g, *Dietary Fiber* 3g, *Sodium* 141mg

Sesame Noodles

Tasty, tangy, and fun to eat, Asian noodles with sesame sauce actually contain peanut butter, which is one of the reasons this dish is so popular. Buckwheat noodles are high in protein. This recipe can even be a great lunch or snack and will keep in the refrigerator for up to one week.

YIELD: 4 SERVINGS

SAUCE

½ cup plain nonfat yogurt

1 teaspoon sesame oil

¼ cup low-sodium soy sauce

1 teaspoon chopped cilantro

¼ cup mirin (Japanese sweet rice wine)

1 teaspoon minced ginger

2 tablespoons reduced-fat peanut butter

⅛ teaspoon Tabasco or other hot pepper sauce

1 tablespoon fructose

1 clove garlic, minced

NOODLES

8 ounces udon noodles (Japanese buckwheat noodles)

1 large carrot, julienned

1 large cucumber, peeled, seeded, and julienned

3 scallions, sliced on the diagonal

¼ cup cilantro, chopped fine

¼ cup dry-roasted soy nuts, chopped

1. For the sauce, combine the yogurt, sesame oil, soy sauce, cilantro, mirin, ginger, peanut butter, Tabasco, fructose, and garlic in a blender and blend until smooth.
2. Cook the noodles according to the package directions and drain well. Add ½ cup of the sauce to the noodles (save the extra sauce for later use). Add the vegetables and toss lightly. Garnish with the cilantro leaves and soy nuts. Serve immediately.

Nutrition Facts:

Serving Size ½ cup, Calories 207, Fat 3g, Saturated Fat 1g, Cholesterol 0mg, Carbohydrate 32g, Protein 10g, Sugars 10g, Dietary Fiber 4g, Sodium 873mg

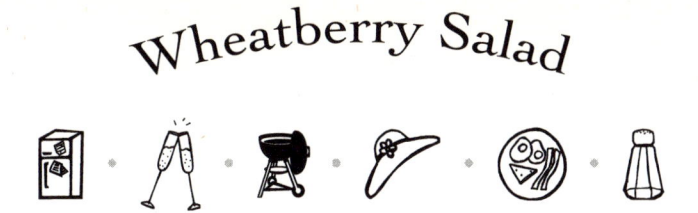

Wheatberry Salad
with Raspberry Vinaigrette

Great to serve cold, this flavorful salad really gives you some substance to dig into with the robust wheatberries and dried cranberries.

YIELD: 6 SERVINGS

SALAD

1 cup wheatberries

1 clove garlic, minced

1 medium onion, peeled and diced fine

1 bay leaf

2 teaspoons dried ground thyme

1 teaspoon grated lemon peel

1 medium carrot chopped

1 stalk celery

½ cup dried cranberries

1 tablespoon chopped parsley

DRESSING

1½ cups raspberries, fresh or frozen

¼ teaspoon ground thyme

¼ teaspoon ground black pepper

2 teaspoons canola oil

1½ teaspoons low-sodium soy sauce

1 tablespoon fructose

1 tablespoon orange juice

1. Simmer the wheatberries in a saucepan with water to cover by 2 inches for 2 minutes. Remove from the heat and let sit for 1 hour. Remove the lid and add enough water to cover by 1 inch.
2. Stir in the garlic, onion, bay leaf, thyme, and lemon peel. Cover and simmer for 45 minutes, until the berries are slightly puffed and softened. Remove from the heat, place in large bowl, and let cool.

3. Peel and cube the carrots. Cut the celery into thin slices. Place the carrots and celery in a medium bowl, add the dried cranberries and parsley, and mix well.
4. To make the dressing, combine the rasberries, thyme, pepper, oil, soy sauce, fructose, and orange juice in a blender or food processor and blend well.
5. Add the cranberry mixture to the wheatberries in a large bowl. Toss with the Raspberry Dressing.
6. Serve and enjoy.

Nutrition Facts:

Serving Size ½ cup, Calories 188, Fat 2g, Saturated Fat 0g, Cholesterol 0mg, Protein 8g, Carbohydrate 38g, Sugars 12g, Dietary Fiber 7g, Sodium 56mg

Gayle's Feel-Good Facts

Wheatberries are also know as groats. They are whole-wheat kernels that have a nutty flavor and chewy texture. They make a hearty, filling side dish.

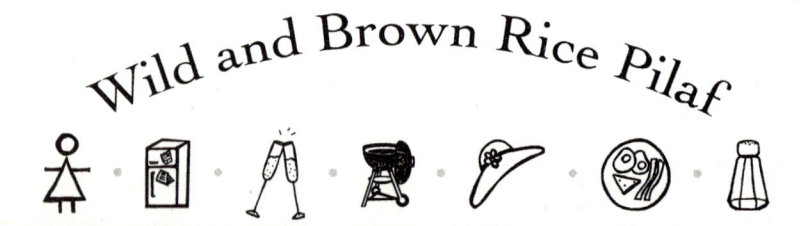

Wild and Brown Rice Pilaf

A great and versatile side for any entrée, it will keep for a week in the refrigerator, or freeze some and defrost for later use.

YIELD: 8 SERVINGS

½ cup yellow onion, finely chopped
½ teaspoon canola oil
1 cup brown rice (long grain)
1 cup wild rice
4 cups water or vegetable broth

1 bunch scallions, sliced diagonally
½ cup chopped parsley
1 teaspoon salt
1 teaspoon black pepper

1. Sauté the onion in the oil. Add the rice and stir to coat with oil. Add the vegetable broth and bring to a boil, then turn down to a simmer.
2. Cover and cook on low heat at a simmer for 30 to 40 minutes, until the broth is absorbed and the rice is tender.
3. When the rice is cooked, stir in the scallions, parsley, salt, and pepper.

Nutrition Facts:

Serving Size ½ cup, *Calories* 40, *Fat* 0g, *Saturated Fat* 0g, *Cholesterol* 0mg, *Protein* 1g, *Carbohydrate* 8g, *Sugars* 1g, *Dietary Fiber* 1g, *Sodium* 295mg

Quick Tip

If you are short on time and don't want to construct your grain side dishes from scratch, feel free to use the preboxed grains that have added seasoning and perk up the flavor with fresh herbs and chopped vegetables or dried fruits when they are finished cooking.

Quinoa with Pesto

This is a simple method for making a grain and adding flavor. You can use this technique anytime with other grains.

YIELD: 4 SERVINGS

2 cups water or vegetable broth

1 cup quinoa, uncooked

½ cup pesto (page 131)

1. Bring the water or vegetable broth to a boil in a medium saucepan. Add the quinoa, cover, reduce heat to low, and simmer for 15 to 20 minutes, until cooked.
2. While the grain is still warm, mix in the pesto and roasted vegetables if desired. Serve warm or at room temperature.

Nutrition Facts:

Serving Size ½ cup, Calories 312, Fat 5g, Saturated Fat 0g, Cholesterol 1mg, Protein 10g, Carbohydrate 47g, Sugars 0g, Dietary Fiber 15g, Sodium 182mg

Gayle's Feel-Good Facts

Quinoa is actually a high-protein seed, not a grain. It was used by the ancient Incas and has now been rediscovered. With 11 grams of protein per half cup, it can be considered a supergrain; it also has higher iron levels than any other grain and a good deal of potassium. Although it is light in texture, it is high in fiber: A perfect healthy accompaniment to any dish.

VEGETABLE SIDES

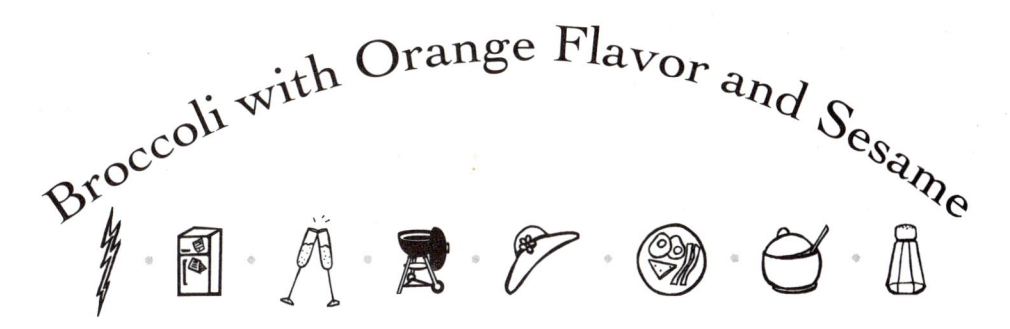

Broccoli with Orange Flavor and Sesame

YIELD: 4 SERVINGS

1 tablespoon olive oil

¾ pound broccoli crowns, cut into medium florets

Zest of 1 orange

½ cup orange juice

4 tablespoons sesame seeds

½ teaspoon salt, optional

1. Heat a large skillet or nonstick wok pan with oil for 2 minutes on high heat. When the pan is hot, add the broccoli florets and zest and stir well. Cook until the broccoli turns a bright green, about 3 to 4 minutes.
2. Turn the heat to medium and add the orange juice. Continue cooking the broccoli until it is tender, about 4 minutes. If the juice evaporates and you need to prevent the broccoli from sticking to the pan, add a bit of water, 1 tablespoon at a time (allow the water to cook off before you add more).
3. When cooked, remove from the pan, sprinkle with sesame seeds and salt if desired. Serve warm, hot, or cold.

Nutrition Facts:

Serving Size 3 ounces broccoli, *Calories* 102, *Fat* 6g, *Saturated Fat* 0g, *Cholesterol* 0mg, *Protein* 4g, *Carbohydrate* 10g, *Sugars* 5g, *Dietary Fiber* 4g, *Sodium* 315mg

Steamed Artichokes in White Wine Broth

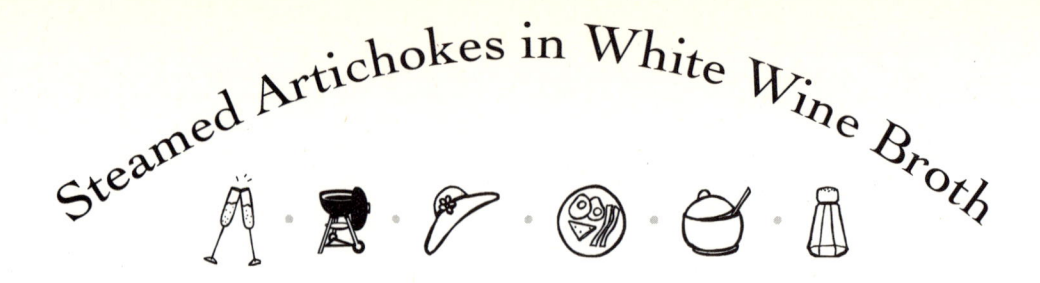

YIELD: 4 SERVINGS

4 medium artichokes	1 medium onion, diced
Juice of 2 lemons	3 small-medium cloves garlic, minced
1½ cups of water	½ teaspoon salt
½ cup dry white wine	¼ teaspoon black pepper
1 tablespoon olive oil	¼ cup grated Parmesan cheese

1. Cut off the artichoke stems and discard. Cut off top ½ inch of artichokes with a serrated knife, then trim ½ inch off all remaining leaf tips with kitchen shears.
2. Squeeze the lemon juice from 1 lemon over the artichokes.
3. To prepare each artichoke — first remove choke, separate the leaves of the artichoke with your thumbs and pull out the purple leaves from the center. You may want to use a spoon to help you dig out the choke. Squeeze some lemon juice into the artichoke after you scoop out the choke.
4. Put the water, wine, oil, onion, garlic, salt, and pepper into a large pot and arrange the artichokes in the water solution.
5. Simmer the artichokes, covered, in the pot for 1 hour, until the leaves are tender.
6. Serve in a bowl with some of the broth on the bottom. Sprinkle each artichoke with Parmesan cheese.
7. Serve with low-fat Caesar dressing on the side from page 117.

Nutrition Facts:

Serving Size 1 artichoke, Calories 178, Fat 5g, Saturated Fat 1g, Cholesterol 23mg, Protein 9g, Carbohydrate 23g, Sugars 7g, Dietary Fiber 9g, Sodium 273mg

Spinach with Indian Spices

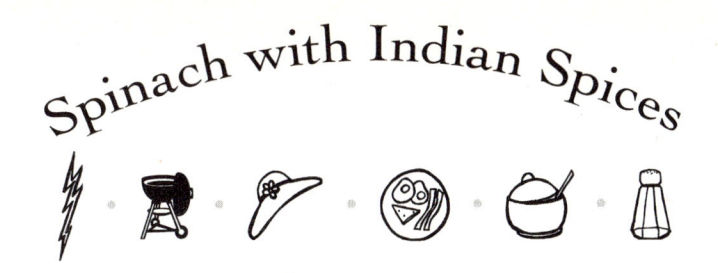

Indian spices are full of flavor and, as in this recipe, are often sautéed to impart a roasted taste to the herbs, prior to using them in a recipe. This recipe calls for cumin and fenugreek, both popular seasonings in Indian cuisine.

YIELD: 4 SERVINGS

2½ tablespoons whole-wheat or all purpose flour

1 cup plain nonfat yogurt

½ teaspoon turmeric

½ teaspoon salt

1 teaspoon canola oil

¼ cup chopped fresh coriander leaves

4 cloves garlic, chopped

½ teaspoon chopped fresh ginger root

1 small onion, chopped

1 tablespoon each cumin seeds and fenugreek seeds

1 pound fresh spinach, chopped

¼ cup water

1. Mix the flour, yogurt, turmeric, and salt with 2 cups of water.
2. Heat a saucepan on medium heat with oil, add the coriander and toast until lightly browned, about 1 minute. Add the chopped garlic, ginger, onion, and cumin and fenugreek seeds. Sauté for 2 minutes. Add the spinach and water and cover to cook for 10 minutes, then add the yogurt mixture.
3. Bring to a boil, then lower to a simmer for 10 minutes. Serve hot.

Nutrition Facts:

Serving Size ½ cup, Calories 158, Fat 2g, Saturated Fat 0g, Cholesterol 1mg, Protein 9g, Carbohydrate 29g, Sugars 5g, Dietary Fiber 2g, Sodium 420mg

Sautéed Greens with Garlic

A nice accompaniment to any Mediterranean style dish.

YIELD: 4 SERVINGS

1 tablespoon olive oil

2 cloves garlic, chopped

1 pound mixed greens (select from spinach, swiss chard, sorrel, and beet greens), washed, trimmed of tough stems, and chopped

½ teaspoon salt

Juice of ½ lemon

1. In a large nonstick sauté pan, heat the oil on medium heat. When the oil is warm, add the garlic and sauté for 2 minutes.
2. Add the chopped mixed greens. Cook on medium heat until wilted. Mix in the salt, and squeeze the lemon juice over all. Mix well and serve.

Nutrition Facts:

Serving Size ½ cup, Calories 50, Fat 3g, Saturated Fat 0g, Cholesterol 0mg, Protein 2g, Carbohydrate 5g, Sugars 0g, Dietary Fiber 2g, Sodium 420mg

Gayle's Feel-Good Facts

Dark green leafy vegetables such as kale, spinach, mustard greens, and broccoli rabe are rich in antioxidants that are protective to your heart. They also contain iron. But the iron is not as available as a dietary source from greens as it is from meat products, which is called heme iron.

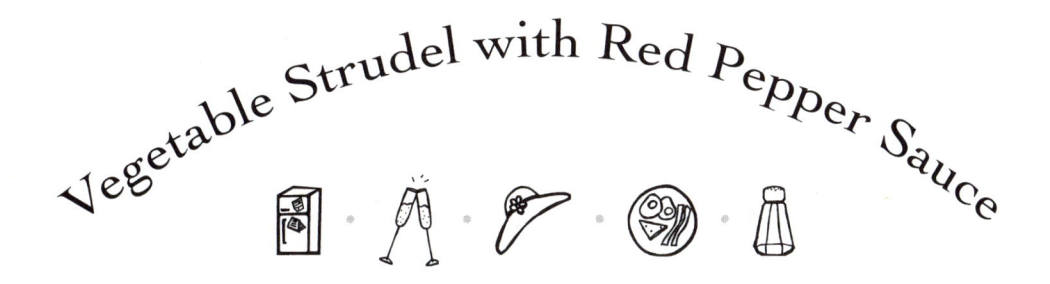

Vegetable Strudel with Red Pepper Sauce

This is a fancier way to serve vegetables and is perfect for a dinner party or as a side or appetizer.

YIELD: 6 SERVINGS

1 large sliced eggplant, peeled, cut into ½-inch strips

1 zucchini, sliced, on the diagonal into ¼-inch pieces

1 red pepper, sliced

1½ teaspoon fresh thyme

1 teaspoon chopped basil

2 teaspoons olive oil

Pinch of salt

1 cup soft low-fat goat cheese

Pinch of black pepper

4 sheets phyllo dough

½ cup drained, wilted spinach

RED PEPPER SAUCE

2 roasted red peppers, sliced in ½-inch wide strips

1 red bell pepper, in ½-inch wide strips

1 garlic clove

Pinch of fructose

¾ cup vegetable broth

Pinch of pepper

Dash of hot sauce or pinch of cayenne

1. In a large bowl combine the eggplant, zucchini, peppers, thyme, basil, oil, and salt. Arrange in a single layer on a baking sheet that has been lined with parchment or foil. Roast all vegetables at 400 degrees for about 8 minutes and then turn them with a spatula. The vegetables are roasted when they are tender and slightly browned. Remove from the oven. Turn the oven down to 375 degrees.
2. In a small bowl mix the goat cheese with the black pepper and set aside.
3. While the vegetables are roasting, prepare the phyllo dough. Place one sheet of phyllo dough on a flat surface, spray with oil spray and lay the second sheet of phyllo dough on top of the first. Continue in the same manner for the third and fourth layers of phyllo dough. When all four layers are together, spread the cheese mixture 1½ inch from the edge of the phyllo dough, spoon spinach over the cheese and then layer the roasted vegetables on top of the spinach.
4. Starting at the long side, roll the phyllo tightly, then roll in the sides of the phyllo slightly to secure the filling. Continue to roll until you form a strudel roll. Seal the end of the roll by spraying it with oil spray.
5. Transfer to a baking sheet lined with foil, seam side down and spray the whole strudel roll lightly with oil spray. Score the top of the strudel through the phyllo, making 6 evenly spaced cuts.
6. Bake the strudel for 30 minutes, or until golden brown.
7. While the strudel is baking prepare the red pepper sauce. Combine the red peppers, garlic clove, fructose, and ¼ cup of the vegetable broth in a medium saucepan and let cook over low heat for 25 minutes. Remove from the heat, remove the garlic, and place in a blender. Purée, adding the remaining broth in increments until the sauce is smooth and the desired consistency. Place back in the saucepan and simmer briefly. Season with black pepper, hot sauce or cayenne. Serve hot over the cooked strudel.

Nutrition Facts:

Serving Size ⅙ *of strudel,* *Calories* 142, *Fat* 5g, *Saturated Fat* 1g, *Cholesterol* 3mg, *Protein* 6g, *Carbohydrate* 21g, *Sugars* 7g, *Dietary Fiber* 4g, *Sodium* 273mg

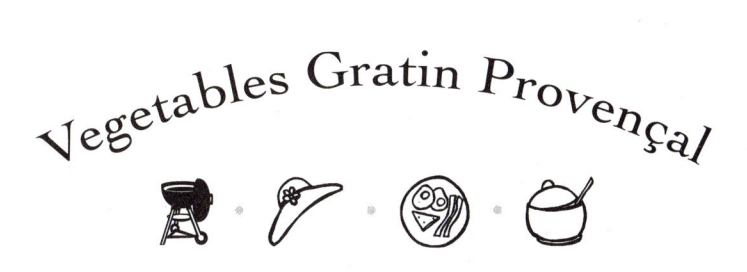

Vegetables Gratin Provençal

YIELD: 6 SERVINGS

- 4 large, ripe tomatoes
- 1 teaspoon canola or olive oil
- 2 large yellow onions, thinly sliced
- 2 cloves garlic, minced
- ¼ cup vegetable broth
- ½ teaspoon dried thyme or 1½ teaspoons fresh
- ½ teaspoon dried oregano or 1½ teaspoons fresh
- 2 medium zucchini or yellow squash, sliced ¼ inch thick
- 1 eggplant, peeled and sliced ¼ inch thick
- ¼ teaspoon salt
- ¼ teaspoon ground black pepper
- ½ cup fresh bread crumbs
- ¼ cup grated imported Parmesan cheese

1. Slice two tomatoes in half and gently cut out the core and seeds; squeeze out the juice and slice the remaining section of the tomato. Cut the other tomatoes into ¼ inch cubes.
2. Heat the oil in a large skillet and add the onions and garlic. Sauté briefly, until the onions are wilted, and then add the broth. Cook until the onions are soft and the liquid has evaporated. Add the cubed tomatoes, thyme, and oregano. Cook for 2 to 3 minutes.
3. Cover the bottom of a gratin dish or shallow baking dish with half of the onion-tomato mixture.

4. Layer the zucchini or squash, sliced tomatoes, and eggplant over the onion mixture. Season with salt and pepper. Top with the rest of the onion mixture. Sprinkle the bread crumbs over the mixture, then top with the Parmesan cheese.
5. Cover with aluminum foil and bake at 375 degrees for 20 minutes. Uncover and bake for 10 to 15 minutes more, or until the top is golden brown and crispy and the mixture is bubbling. Serve warm.

Nutrition Facts:

Serving Size ½ cup, Calories 110, Fat 3g, Saturated Fat 1g, Cholesterol 3mg, Protein 5g, Carbohydrate 18g, Sugars 5g, Dietary Fiber 3g, Sodium 150mg

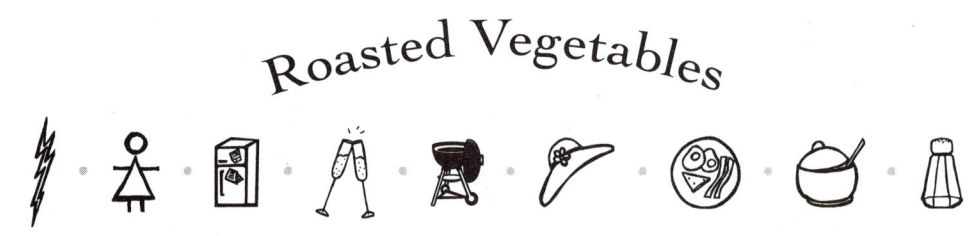

Roasted Vegetables

Roasting vegetables brings out their sweetness. I find this a very satisfying way to have vegetables. This recipe allows you to roast many vegetables all at once.

YIELD: 6 SERVINGS

1 red bell pepper, cored, seeded, and cut into strips

1 yellow bell pepper, cored, seeded, and cut into strips

2 red onions, peeled and cut into wedges

2 small summer yellow squash, ends trimmed, cut into ½-inch thick strips

2 small zucchini, ends trimmed, cut into ½-inch thick strips

4 cloves garlic, thinly sliced

1 tablespoon olive oil

1 tablespoon chopped oregano

1 teaspoon salt

Freshly ground black pepper to taste

2 tablespoons chopped parsley

1 tablespoon balsamic vinegar

1. In a large bowl, toss together the peppers, onions, squash, zucchini, garlic, olive oil, oregano, salt, and pepper.
2. Spread the vegetables on a baking sheet or metal roasting pan and roast at 450 degrees for 20 minutes, or until tender, stirring several times.
3. Transfer to a serving bowl and cool slightly. Add the parsley and vinegar and toss until mixed. Taste and adjust seasoning.
4. Serve hot or room temperature.

Nutrition Facts:

Serving Size 1 cup, *Calories* 67, *Fat* 3g, *Saturated Fat* 0g, *Cholesterol* 0mg, *Protein* 2g, *Carbohydrate* 11g, *Sugars* 6g, *Dietary Fiber* 3g, *Sodium* 393mg

9

Desserts

Everyone deserves a sweet treat. When you are trying to eat healthy or watch your blood sugar level, the key to enjoying a tasty dessert is to make sure it is low-fat and a limited portion. The recipes I have listed here give you the satisfaction of rich desserts without the guilt.

Because sweets make you crave more sweets, be sure to have your dessert after a meal and the meal will act as a buffer to slow down the rate at which your body absorbs the sugar from the dessert. So, relax and enjoy the recipes in this section. They are fun to make and eat!

Apple Crisp

A quick, low-fat version of this healthy treat, you can make this individually or in a large baking dish. Use this all-purpose topping for other fruits such as pears, peaches, berries, or rhubarb. Dried cherries or cranberries make a flavorful addition. I like to prepare this dessert ahead of time and have it handy for an easy after-dinner treat during the week.

YIELD: 4 SERVINGS

FILLING	TOPPING
4 large apples	¼ cup walnuts
1 tablespoon fresh lemon juice	2 tablespoons whole-wheat flour
1 teaspoon cinnamon	2 tablespoons dark brown sugar
2 tablespoons maple syrup	2 teaspoons ground cinnamon
1 tablespoon all-purpose flour (optional)	1 tablespoon butter
	2 cups (12 ounce/350g) low-fat granola
	1 egg white

1. Preheat the oven to 375° F. To make the filling, peel and core the apples and dice. Toss the apple pieces with the lemon juice, cinnamon, maple syrup, and flour, if using. Spread the mixture evenly in 4 individual ramekins or in a shallow gratin dish.
2. To make the topping, combine the nuts, flour, brown sugar, cinnamon, butter, and granola in a food processor and pulse briefly. Add the egg white, a little at a time, until the mixture starts to clump. Do not let the mixture get too wet or it will turn soggy.
3. Using your hands, spread the topping over the apples. Bake 15 minutes, or until the apples are simmering and the topping is brown and crisp. Cool slightly before serving.

Nutrition Facts:

Serving Size ¼ crisp, Calories 238, Fat 3g, Saturated Fat 1g, Cholesterol 8mg, Carbohydrate 42g, Protein 1g, Sugars 38g, Dietary Fiber 5g, Sodium 52mg

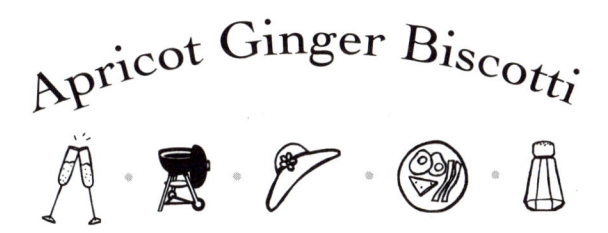

Apricot Ginger Biscotti

This cookie will satisfy your desire for crunch and sweet without a lot of calories.

YIELD: 12 SERVINGS

2 eggs

½ cup sugar

1⅓ cups flour

¼ teaspoon baking soda

¼ teaspoon baking powder

¼ teaspoon salt

½ teaspoon vanilla

⅓ cup dried apricots, chopped

3 tablespoons crystallized ginger, chopped

1. Combine the eggs and sugar in a small mixing bowl and set aside.
2. Blend the flour, baking soda and powder, and salt. Add the egg mixture and vanilla.
3. Mix in the apricots and ginger.
4. With floured hands, form the dough into a 6½-x-4½-inch rectangle.
5. Bake at 325 degrees for 30 minutes. Take out and slice on a diagonal.
6. Lay the cut biscotti on the baking sheet on their flat side and rebake for 10 minutes.
7. Remove and let cool. Serve.

Nutrition Facts:

Serving Size 1 biscotti, *Calories* 64, *Fat* 1g, *Saturated Fat* 0g, *Cholesterol* 31mg, *Protein* 1g, *Carbohydrate* 13g, *Sugars* 10g, *Dietary Fiber* 0g, *Sodium* 90mg

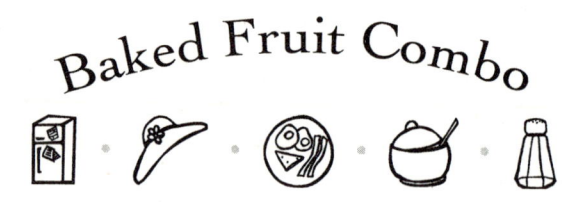

Baked Fruit Combo

A great way to get in your fruit. This dish is particularly satisfying on a cold day. Feel free to serve it with low-fat frozen yogurt on the side.

YIELD: 6 SERVINGS

2 ripe pears (Anjou or Bartlett)

2 Granny Smith or Golden Delicious apples

4 small ripe apricots, cut into ½-inch slices

4 small ripe plums, cut into ½-inch slices

1 tablespoon orange juice

1 tablespoon lemon juice

1 tablespoon unsalted butter

1 tablespoon apricot preserves

¾ cup water

1. Peel, halve, and core the pears. Peel, core, and quarter the apples. Cut the apricots and plums into quarters.
2. Place the pears flat side down in a gratin or small casserole dish. Arrange the apple slices around the pears and cover with the apricots and plums. Sprinkle with orange and lemon juice and add the water. Dot with the butter and then spoon the preserves on top.
3. Bake at 400 degrees for 35 to 45 minutes, adding a little water so it doesn't burn or get too dry.
4. Let cool slightly and serve with vanilla fat-free yogurt (frozen or fresh).

Nutrition Facts:

Serving size ½ cup, Calories 110, Fat 3g, Saturated Fat 1g, Cholesterol 5mg, Protein 1g, Carbohydrate 24g, Dietary Fiber 3g, Sugars 17g, Sodium 2mg

Gayle's Feel-Good Facts

Apricots are packed with carotenes, vitamin C, and potassium. Recent research has shown we are not getting enough potassium in our diets. Enjoy eating this dessert and think about all you are giving your body at the same time.

Banana Bread Pudding

Most people love bananas and pudding, this recipe puts them together for a sweet treat. Children will like this recipe too.

YIELD: 8 SERVINGS

- 4 cups cubed wheat bread
- 1 tablespoon fructose
- 2 large eggs
- ¾ cup plus 2 tablespoons dark brown sugar
- 2 cups evaporated skim milk
- 1 tablespoon vanilla extract
- 1½ teaspoons cinnamon
- ½ teaspoon nutmeg
- 2 bananas, sliced
- 1 teaspoon butter, melted

1. Toast the bread cubes until light brown . Spray either a 2-quart baking dish or 8 individual ramekins with oil spray and sprinkle with ½ tablespoon of the fructose.
2. In a medium mixing bowl, whisk together the eggs and brown sugar. Blend in the milk vanilla, and spices.
3. Stir the bread cubes into the egg mixture. Cover and refrigerate for 1 hour.
4. Mix the sliced bananas into the bread mixture and pour into the prepared dish. Drizzle melted butter and remaining fructose on top. Bake at 325 degrees for 40 minutes. Increase the temperature to 425 and bake 10 minutes longer, until the pudding is puffy. Let cool. Serve hot or at room temperature.

Nutrition Facts:

Serving Size 1 cup, *Calories* 232, *Fat* 3g, *Saturated Fat* 1g, *Cholesterol* 57mg, *Protein* 10g, *Carbohydrate* 42g, *Sugars* 28g, *Dietary Fiber* 3g, *Sodium* 245mg

Gayle's Feel-Good Facts

Pudding is a good way to help your children take in their needed calcium. Most people, children included, do not take in enough calcium to build strong bones. In general, most people should consume either three servings of foods high in calcium, which include 8 ounces of yogurt, 8 ounces of skim milk, ½ cup part skim ricotta, and parmesan cheese.

Banana Rum Parfait

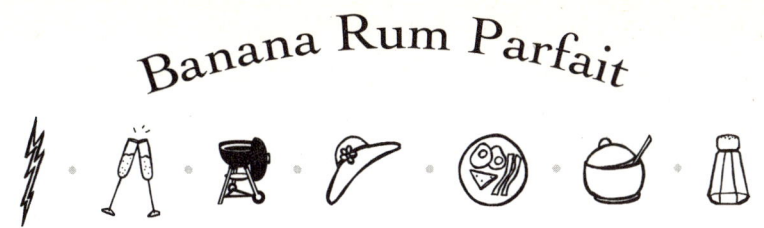

A taste of the Caribbean anytime, this is a delightful way to add pizzazz to frozen yogurt.

YIELD: 4 SERVINGS

2 tablespoons brown sugar

½ teaspoon ginger, ground

3 tablespoons Jamaican rum

4 bananas, sliced on the diagonal, ½ inch thick

4 tablespoons fat-free caramel ice cream sauce

2 cups vanilla low-fat or fatfree frozen yogurt

¼ cup chopped hazelnuts, toasted

4 gingersnaps

1. Mix together the brown sugar, ginger, and rum.
2. Spray a nonstick medium skillet and heat on low-medium heat. Add the banana slices and brown sugar and rum mixture. Sauté until they are just cooked and slightly caramelized, about 4 to 6 minutes. Set aside.
3. Heat the caramel sauce according to package directions.
4. Scoop ½ cup of vanilla frozen yogurt into 4 parfait or ice cream dishes. Pour the warm caramel sauce over the ice cream. Divide the bananas equally among 4 servings and sprinkle hazelnuts on top. Place a gingersnap on the side. Serve right away.

Nutrition Facts:

Serving Size ½ cup, Calories 378, Fat 8g, Saturated Fat 2g, Cholesterol 7.5mg, Protein 7g, Carbohydrate 70g, Sugars 61g, Dietary Fiber 3g, Sodium 178mg

Blueberry Cobbler

Traditionally made with butter, this low-fat version uses nonfat sour cream to create the richness and moistness in the topping.

YIELD: 4 SERVINGS

3 cups blueberries

½ teaspoon grated orange zest

¼ cup plus 2 tablespoons nonfat sour cream

1 tablespoon honey

2 egg whites

3 tablespoons nonfat milk

1 tablespoon butter, melted

2 tablespoons fructose

½ cup whole-wheat or whole-grain flour

½ teaspoon baking powder

Pinch of salt

1. Preheat the oven to 350 degrees.
2. In a medium bowl, gently mix the blueberries, zest, sour cream, and honey. Spoon the berries into 4 ½-cup ramekins.
3. In a small bowl, beat the egg whites lightly with a fork. Stir in the milk, butter, remaining 2 tablespoons of sour cream, and fructose.
4. In another small bowl, combine the flour, baking powder, and salt. Add the flour mixture to the egg mixture and mix until just blended.
5. Spoon 2 tablespoons of the batter on top of the blueberries. Place the ramekins on a baking sheet and bake for 15 to 20 minutes, or until the tops are golden brown.

Nutrition Facts:

Serving Size ¼ cobbler, Calories 198, Fat 4g, Saturated Fat 2g, Cholesterol 9mg, Protein 5g, Carbohydrate 38g, Sugars 22g, Dietary Fiber 5g, Sodium 150mg

Gayle's Feel-Good Facts

I have used fructose instead of sugar in most of the recipes because fructose is sweeter than sugar, so you can use less. Also, it doesn't raise your blood sugars as high as fast, so you are less likely to crave more sweets after eating something with fructose.

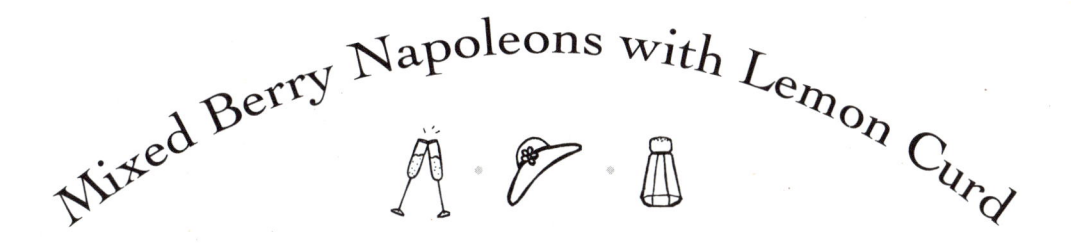

Mixed Berry Napoleons with Lemon Curd

An elegant party or special dinner dessert. It is easy to make. Just follow the directions step by step.

YIELD: 4 SERVINGS

- 3 phyllo leaves, 14-x-18 inches
- oil spray
- 3 teaspoons granulated sugar
- 1/4 cup unsalted raw, shelled pistachios, finely chopped
- 1 1/2 cups fresh mixed berries (strawberries [chopped], blueberries, raspberries)
- 1 1/2 cups Lemon Curd (see recipe under Lemon Tart, page 243)
- 2 tablespoons of powdered sugar
- Raspberry Coulis (optional) (page 237)

1. Defrost phyllo according to package directions.
2. Line a baking sheet with parchment paper. Have a second baking sheet on hand that is the same size. Spread one of the phyllo leaves on a sheet and spray with

oil spray or brush lightly with canola oil, making sure to brush edges so they don't dry out.

3. Sprinkle one-third of the sugar over the phyllo and then one-third of the ground nuts. Place a second phyllo leaf on top, lightly press down around the edges and center of dough and repeat the procedure. Repeat again for the third layer. Spray the top of the third layer with oil spray or lightly brush with oil. With a sharp knife, cut the leaves into 12 equal squares.

4. To cook, place a piece of parchment paper on top of the phyllo and cover with the second baking sheet so that the phyllo dough is firmly sandwiched between the two baking sheets. Bake at 375 degrees for 7 to 8 minutes, or until the leaves are golden brown and crisp. Remove the top baking sheet and let the phyllo cool.

5. Wash and pick over the berries.

6. To serve: place one square on each of the serving plates. Add about 3 tablespoons of Lemon Curd and 2 to 3 tablespoons of berries. Stack another square on top and add more curd. Top with a final phyllo square and sift powdered sugar over the top. Decorate the plate with the Raspberry Coulis if desired by either spooning the sauce around the sides of the napoleon or placing the sauce in a squeeze bottle and dotting the edges of the plate.

Nutrition Facts:

Serving Size 1 Napolean, *Calories* 312, *Fat* 6g, *Saturated Fat* 0g, *Cholesterol* 53mg, *Protein* 5g, *Carbohydrate* 64g, *Sugars* 18g, *Dietary Fiber* 2g, *Sodium* 87mg

Raspberry Coulis

A great sauce to keep on hand. It can be used for decoration on the plate. Using a squeeze bottle, you can make designs with the sauce. All designs on a plate should be eatable. You can also use the Raspberry Coulis as a sauce for frozen yogurt or low-fat ice cream. It will keep in the refrigerator for a week and the freezer for at least 6 months.

YIELD: 1 CUP (16 SERVINGS)

2 cups fresh or frozen raspberries, thawed

1 tablespoon lemon juice

¼ to ½ cup confectioners' sugar (depending on sweetness of berries)

1. Puree all ingredients in a blender until very smooth.
2. Strain through a fine strainer to remove any seeds.
3. Refrigerate or use for desired desserts.

Nutrition Facts:

Serving Size 1 tablespoon, *Calories* 15, *Fat* 0g, *Saturated Fat* 0g, *Cholesterol* 0mg, *Protein* 0g, *Carbohydrate* 4g, *Sugars* 3g, *Dietary Fiber* 1g, *Sodium* 0mg

Fruit Salad with Yogurt Honey Lime Dressing

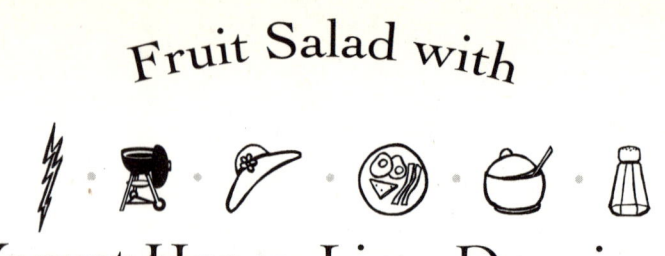

The freshness of the honey and lime really helps to bring out the sweet taste of the fruits in this colorful, tasty fruit salad.

YIELD: 12 SERVINGS

4 large golden pineapples

1 large honeydew

1 large cantaloupe

4 oranges

4 pints strawberries

¾ cup fresh mint leaves (optional), chiffonade

YOGURT HONEY LIME DRESSING

2 cups fat-free plain yogurt

4 tablespoons honey

4 tablespoons lime juice

1 teaspoon lime zest

1. Cut the pineapples and melons into cubes.
2. Slice the berries in half.
3. Peel and cut two oranges into segments.
4. Mix all the fruit together in a large bowl. Squeeze the juice of the remaining two oranges onto the fruit.
5. In a medium bowl, mix together all the dressing ingredients. Serve on the side or coat the fruit salad with the dressing just before serving.
6. Sprinkle the mint on top and serve.

Nutrition Facts:

Serving Size 1 cup, Calories 228, Fat 1g, Saturated Fat 0g, Cholesterol 0mg, Protein 5g, Carbohydrate 60g, Sugars 47g, Dietary Fiber 8g, Sodium 46mg

> ### Gayle's Feel-Good Facts
>
> Yogurt contains live bacteria cultures which keep your digestive system in good health.

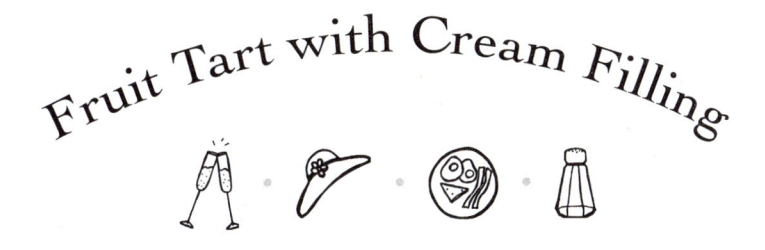

Fruit Tart with Cream Filling

For all those who forgo cream fillings, this is a great way to have it, with fruit to keep the calories down and add sweetness. For a large tart, you can use a frozen piecrust that has been thawed. And for cream, you can use the low-fat or skim milk pre-made pudding to fill the tart. You can also make these tarts miniature by putting the cream filling into Athens mini phyllo tart shells, which you can find in your freezer case at the supermarket. Follow the directions on the mini tart shells to prebake, then just add the cream and top with fruit. On the mini tarts, you may want to just top with berries, since the tarts are so small.

YIELD: 10 SERVINGS

1 frozen pie shell (Pet Ritz is a recommended brand)

1 egg yolk

2 tablespoons sugar

1 teaspoon vanilla

1 tablespoon cornstarch

1 cup low-fat milk

FRUIT TOPPINGS

½ cup blueberries

¼ cup strawberries, sliced thin

2 peaches, sliced in ¼-inch slices

½ cup apricot preserves

1. Spray an 8-inch tart pan with removable base or tart baking dish with oil spray. Thaw the pie shell and transfer it to the tart pan. Crimp the edges with your finger to form a border.
2. In a medium bowl, whisk together the egg yolk, sugar, vanilla, and cornstarch. Set aside.
3. In a small saucepan bring the milk to a boil and then turn the heat down to medium-high. Add some hot milk to the egg mixture and whisk well. Add the hot egg mixture to the remainder of the hot milk and mix to combine in the saucepan. Whisk the milk-egg mixture constantly over medium-high heat for one minute, until it thickens. If you would like it thicker, make a slurry with 1 teaspoon of cornstarch and water and add to the cream mixture while stirring.
4. Transfer the cream to a large bowl to cool to room temperature, cover, and refrigerate until cool.
5. Clean the fruit and heat the apricot preserves in a small pan until simmering, or in the microwave for 1 minute. When the cream is cooled, place the cream in the tart shell, then decorate the tops with the fruit. Using a pastry brush, brush the top with the apricot preserves to give the fruit a shiny coating. Serve cold.

Nutrition Facts:

Serving Size ⅛ tart, Calories 195, Fat 5g, Saturated Fat 2g, Cholesterol 34mg, Protein 3g, Carbohydrate 36g, Sugars 21g, Dietary Fiber 1g, Sodium 121mg

Glazed Venetian Oranges

Display this beautiful fruit in glass dishes and wait to hear the oos and aahs.

YIELD: 10 SERVINGS

10 navel or blood oranges

2 cups sugar

1 cup orange juice

¼ cup lemon juice

1 cinnamon stick

1 cup water

½ cup liquor (rum, kirsch, or Grand Marnier)

½ cup pistachios, chopped (optional)

10 to 15 fresh mint leaves (optional)

1. Using a vegetable peeler, peel the oranges, taking as little of the white pith as possible. With a sharp knife peel the oranges of all the white pith. This keeps the orange as round as possible. Cut a slice off the bottom of each orange so it can sit on a flat side.
2. Julienne the orange peel into very thin slivers.
3. In a nonreactive sauce pan that will hold all the oranges in one layer, boil the sugar, juices, peels, cinnamon stick, and water gently for about 6 to 8 minutes.
4. Add the oranges and cook gently for another 5 minutes, turning them to coat in the syrup. Remove the cinnamon stick. Remove the oranges and add the liquor of your choice and turn off the heat. Place the oranges in a baking dish and pour the syrup over them. Put in the refrigerator to cool.
5. To serve, pour the sauce over the tops of the oranges. You can also sprinkle chopped pistachios on the orange or decorate with mint leaves.

Nutrition Facts:

Serving Size 1 *orange, Calories* 179, *Fat* 0g, *Saturated Fat* 0g, *Cholesterol* 0mg, *Protein* 2g, *Carbohydrate* 48g, *Sugars* 31g, *Dietary Fiber* 7g, *Sodium* 4mg

Pistachios per serving add: Calories 37, *Fat* 3g, *Saturated Fat* 0g, *Cholesterol* 0mg *Protein* 1g, *Carbohydrate* 2g, *Sugars* 0g, *Dietary Fiber* 0g, *Sodium* 0mg

Homemade Fat-Free Chocolate Pudding

A comfort food recipe for those cold nights, or anytime you want to curl up on the couch with a tasty dessert.

YIELD: 4 SERVINGS

2 cups skim milk

3 tablespoons cornstarch

½ cup good-quality unsweetened cocoa powder

¼ teaspoon cinnamon

½ cup sugar

1 teaspoon vanilla extract

Pinch of salt (optional)

1. Place 1½ cups of the milk in a heavy saucepan. Heat until almost boiling.
2. Combine the cornstarch, cocoa, cinnamon, and sugar.
3. Whisk in the remaining ½ cup of milk until smooth. Add the mixture to the hot milk.
4. Cook, stirring over medium heat, until smooth and thick.
5. Add the vanilla and salt if desired, stir, and remove from heat.
6. Pour into four small serving bowls and chill. (If you want, place wax paper directly on the surface while cooling to prevent a skin from forming.)

Nutrition Facts:

Serving Size ½ cup, Calories 195, Fat 2g, Saturated Fat 1g, Cholesterol 2mg, Protein 43g, Carbohydrate 42g, Sugars 30g, Dietary Fiber 0g, Sodium 138mg

Lemon Tart

This is a great dessert to serve or bring to someone's house, because it's colorful, elegant, and no one will know it is low-fat, unless you want them to.

YIELD: 18 SERVINGS

1 frozen piecrust, thawed
2 tablespoon confectioners' sugar
3/4 cup sugar or fructose
1 tablespoon plus 2 teaspoons cornstarch
5 teaspoons grated lemon zest

1/2 cup water
1/3 cup fresh lemon juice
2 drops yellow food coloring (optional)
1 egg, lightly beaten
1/2 cup raspberries

1. Remove the piecrust from the aluminum pan and press into a 9-inch tart shell that has been sprayed or lightly coated with oil.
2. Sprinkle the bottom and sides of the piecrust with 2 teaspoons of confectioners' sugar. Using a fork, make several pricks into the bottom of the crust to help avoid air bubbles.
3. Bake the tart shell in a 350-degree oven for 25 minutes, until the top of the shell looks firm and light brown. Cool on a wire rack.
4. In a medium saucepan, combine the sugar, cornstarch, and lemon zest. Mix well.
5. Gradually add the water and lemon juice; stir with a whisk until well blended.
6. Bring to a boil over medium heat; cook 1 minute, stirring constantly.
7. Gradually stir a small portion of the hot lemon mixture into the egg to temper. Add the egg mixture to the lemon mixture, stirring constantly.
8. Add the food coloring, if desired, and cook over medium heat until thickened, about 1 minute. Add more cornstarch if mixture is too loose. Simply mix 1 teaspoon of cornstorch with water, stir into lemon mixture, and bring to a boil to thicken.

9. Remove from the heat and pour into the tart shell. Allow to cool to room temperature, then place in the refrigerator to chill.
10. Decorate the finished tart with fresh raspberries around the sides and in the middle. Sift the remaining teaspoon of confectioner's sugar over the top of the tart and serve.

Nutrition Facts:

Serving Size 1/8 *tart, Calories* 108, *Fat* 1g, *Saturated Fat* 0g, *Cholesterol* 24mg, *Protein* 1g, *Carbohydrate* 24g, *Sugars* 20g, *Dietary Fiber* 0g, *Sodium* 15mg

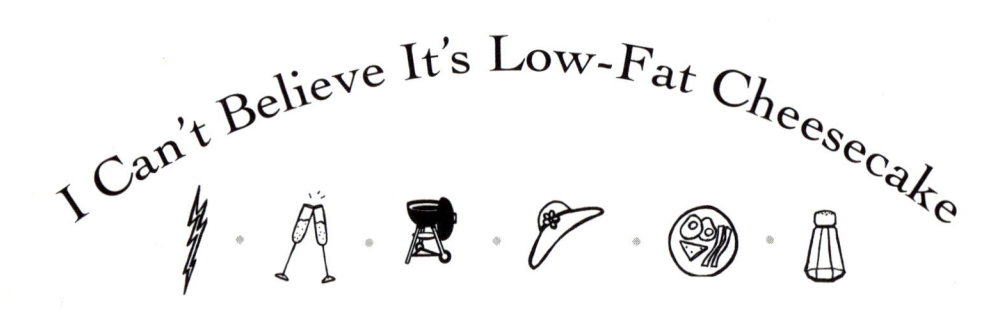

I Can't Believe It's Low-Fat Cheesecake

A favorite among my friends and family. This is easy to make as you do most of the work in the food processor.

YIELD: 10 SERVINGS

CRUST

1 1/2 cups graham cracker crumbs

CHEESECAKE

2 8-ounce packages low-fat cream cheese

1 cup sugar

1 8-ounce container egg substitute or 8 egg whites

2 tablespoons fresh lemon juice

2 teaspoons grated lemon zest

1 1/2 teaspoons pure vanilla extract

1/4 teaspoon salt

1 pound fat-free or low-fat sour cream

244

TOPPING

12 ounces dried California apricots

1¼ cups water

½ cup sugar

2 teaspoons Grand Marnier or other orange liqueur

1 teaspoon orange juice

1. Spray an 8-inch springform pan with cooking oil spray. Coat the bottom of the pan with the graham cracker crumbs.
2. In a food processor or with an electric mixer, beat the cream cheese and sugar until very smooth, about 3 minutes. Blend in the egg substitute or egg whites.
3. Add the lemon juice, zest, vanilla, and salt. Blend until well mixed. Beat in the sour cream, just until blended.
4. Pour the batter into the prepared pan. Wrap the bottom of the pan with foil to prevent leakage. Set the pan in a larger pan and surround it with 1 inch of very hot water. Bake at 350 degrees for 45 minutes, or until firm in center. Turn off the oven without opening the door and let the cake set for 1 hour.
5. To make the topping, place the apricots and water in a saucepan, cover tightly, and simmer for 20 minutes over medium heat until the apricots are soft. Add the sugar and Grand Marnier and simmer for 5 more minutes. Puree the mixture in a food processor or blender. Press through a fine strainer. Stir in the orange juice. Spread the topping over the cheesecake and refrigerate.
6. When ready to serve, run a thin metal spatula around the sides of the cake and release the sides of the springform pan.

Nutrition Facts

Serving Size ¹⁄₁₀ cake, *Calories* 181, *Fat* 2g, *Saturated Fat* 0g, *Cholesterol* 0mg, *Carbohydrate* 92g, *Protein* 8g, *Sugars* 46g, *Dietary Fiber* 2g, *Sodium* 304mg

Quick Tip

If you are short on time or want to save on calories, you can omit the apricot topping and use canned lite cherry or blueberry pie filling for the top of the cake.

Low-Fat Fudge Brownie

The better the quality of chocolate and cocoa powder, the better the brownie. Some excellent quality cocoa powders include Ghirardelli, Droste, Callebaut, or Scharfenberger.

YIELD: 9 BROWNIES

1 1/3 cups all purpose unbleached flour

1 1/4 cups confectioners' sugar

1/2 cup unsweetened cocoa powder

1 teaspoon baking powder

Pinch of salt

2 ounces bittersweet chocolate, coarsely chopped

2 teaspoons canola oil

2 teaspoons unsalted butter

4 tablespoons light corn syrup

2 teaspoons pure vanilla extract

4 large egg whites

1. Line an 8-inch square baking pan with aluminum foil. Spray with cooking oil spray.
2. In a medium bowl, sift together the flour, sugar, cocoa, baking powder, and salt.
3. In a heavy, medium saucepan, combine the chocolate, oil, and butter and heat over very low heat, stirring until melted and smooth. Do not let the chocolate burn.
4. Remove from the heat and stir in the corn syrup and vanilla. Mix the egg whites.
5. Stir the dry ingredients into the chocolate mixture until the batter is smooth and dense. Transfer the batter to the prepared baking pan and spread evenly. Bake at 350 degrees for 20 minutes, or until the center top is almost firm.
6. Cool on a wire rack. Remove the foil from the pan and peel off of the bottom of the brownies.
7. Cut the brownies into 9 bars, trimming off the edges if dry. Store in an airtight container or wrap each one in plastic wrap and refrigerate.

Nutrition Facts:

Serving Size 1 brownie, *Calories* 255, *Fat* 3g, *Saturated Fat* 1.5g, *Cholesterol* 0mg, *Carbohydrate* 36g, *Protein* 2g, *Sugars* 18g, *Dietary Fiber* 0g, *Sodium* 50mg

---

Gayle's Feel-Good Facts

Cocoa powder contains antioxidants called flavanols, which help reduce blood pressure.

Low-Fat Rugelach

This recipe takes a bit more time, but if you like mini pastries, it is worth it.

YIELD: 15 SERVINGS

- 2 cups white flour
- 2 tablespoons sugar
- ¼ teaspoon salt
- 8 ounces low-fat cream cheese
- 4 ounces low-fat sour cream
- 2 tablespoons butter

- 1 cup currants
- 1 tablespoon cornstarch
- ½ cup cinnamon
- ½ cup fructose
- 1 egg
- 1 tablespoon milk

FILLING

- 1½ cups diced apple
- 1 cup chopped dried cranberry

1. Pulse the flour, sugar, and salt in a food processor. Add cream cheese and pulse until the mixture is like coarse meal.
2. Add the sour cream and butter. Pulse until loose and sticky but not overblended. Roll the dough into a thick log and cut into 4 sections. Flatten the sections and roll with a rolling pin in-between plastic wrap to form 4 rectangles, ¼-inch thick by 6 inches long. Refrigerate for at least 30 minutes. This dough can be made ahead.
3. Combine the apple, cranberry, currants, and cornstarch in a strainer over a medium bowl to remove extra liquid from the apples.
4. Combine the cinnamon and fructose in a small bowl.
5. In a separate small bowl, combine the egg and milk.
6. On a floured surface, roll out the dough into thin, long strips.
7. Sprinkle the dough with the cinnamon mixture and then dried fruit mixture. Spread the filling evenly and roll widthwise. Brush the top of the rugelah with the egg mixture and sprinkle the top of the pastry with cinnamon and fructose.
8. Slice into 2-inch cookies. Line a baking sheet with parchment paper. Bake for 15 to 20 minutes at 350 degrees. Remove the cookies to a cooling rack and let cool. Serve.

Nutrition Facts:

Serving Size 1 piece, *Calories* 48, *Fat* 2g, *Saturated Fat* 0g, *Cholesterol* 3mg, *Protein* 0g, *Carbohydrate* 9g, *Sugar* 19g, *Dietary Fiber* 0g, *Sodium* 93mg.

Gayle's Feel-Good Facts

Cinnamon is a warm spice that has been used medicinally to relieve nausea and indigestion.

Oatmeal Chocolate Chip Cookies

Everyone loves a good chocolate chip cookie. This one is packed with oats, so it also has a good amount of fiber.

YIELD: 2 DOZEN

2 tablespoons butter	½ cup all-purpose flour
2 tablespoons canola oil	¼ cup whole-wheat or whole-grain flour
½ cup fructose	1½ cups old-fashioned rolled oats
⅓ cup brown sugar	1 teaspoon baking soda
1 egg	¼ teaspoon salt
½ cup sweetened applesauce	3 ounces miniature semi-sweet chocolate chips
1 teaspoon vanilla extract	½ cup walnuts, chopped fine (optional)

1. Preheat the oven to 350 degrees. Spray the cookie sheets with nonstick vegetable spray or line with foil and set aside.
2. In a large bowl, cream the butter and oil with the fructose and brown sugar. Add the egg and mix well. Add the applesauce and vanilla. Mix well and set aside.
3. In a medium bowl, combine the flours, oats, baking soda, and salt. Add to the creamed mixture and mix well. Add the chocolate chips and walnuts if desired.
4. Using a tablespoon, spoon the dough onto the prepared baking sheet, spacing them about 1 inch apart. Bake for 8 to 10 minutes, until the cookies are golden.
5. They may be a bit soft in the center, but the sides should be cooked. Remove from the oven and transfer to a wire rack. They will firm up further as they cool.

Nutrition Facts:

Serving Size 1 cookie, *Calories* 105, *Fat* 3g, *Saturated Fat* 1g, *Cholesterol* 11mg, *Protein* 2g, *Carbohydrate* 14g, *Sugars* 8g, *Dietary Fiber* 0g, *Sodium* 82mg
Walnuts add: Calories 16, *Fat* 1g

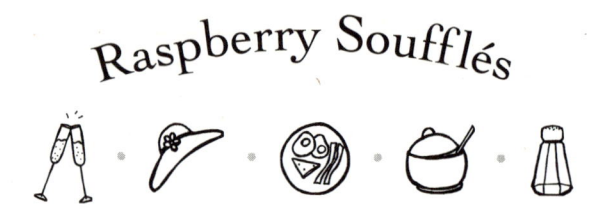

Raspberry Soufflés

Elegant and light, this soufflé is worth making.

YIELD: 6 SERVINGS

- ¾ cup plus 2 tablespoons sugar, divided
- 2 10-ounce packages frozen raspberries in syrup
- 1 tablespoon cornstarch
- 4 large eggs, separated
- 2 tablespoons Framboise liqueur
- ½ teaspoon vanilla extract
- ¼ teaspoon cream of tartar
- ⅛ teaspoon salt
- 1 teaspoon powdered sugar

1. Coat six 8-ounce ramekins with cooking spray and sprinkle each dish with 2 teaspoons of the sugar.
2. Remove 36 raspberries from the bag and drain on paper towels to remove excess moisture. In a small saucepan stir together the remaining raspberries with the syrup with the cornstarch over medium heat. Simmer the mixture until it thickens, about 3 minutes. Pour the raspberry mixture through a fine sieve into a bowl. Stir in the reserved raspberries. Cool.
3. Place the egg yolks in a large bowl; beat with a mixer at medium-high speed for 5 minutes, or until thick and pale. Gradually add ¼ cup of the granulated sugar

and beat a few minutes longer, until light yellow and well combined. Add the Framboise liqueur, raspberry mixture, and vanilla extract.

4. In another bowl with cleaned beaters, beat the egg whites until frothy, add the cream of tartar and salt until they form stiff peaks. Add the remaining 2 tablespoons of sugar until stiff glossy peaks form.

5. Using a large rubber spatula, fold one-third of the egg whites into the raspberry mixture to lighten it up, then fold the remaining whites gently but thoroughly.

6. Divide the soufflé mixture among the ramekins and smooth the tops with a knife. Bake at 375 degrees on a baking sheet in the lower third of the oven until puffed and golden brown, 18 to 20 minutes. Sprinkle with powdered sugar and serve immediately. If you would like to use Raspberry Coulis (page 237) to decorate the plate, this can add a festive touch.

Nutrition Facts:

Serving Size 1 soufflé, *Calories* 150, *Fat* 3g, *Saturated Fat* 0g, *Cholesterol* 142mg, *Protein* 5g, *Carbohydrate* 25g, *Sugars* 18g, *Dietary Fiber* 6g, *Sodium* 90mg

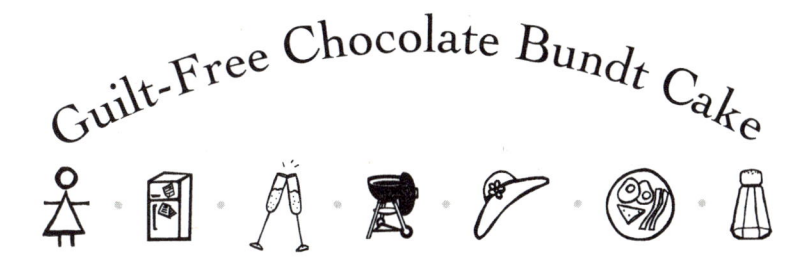

Guilt-Free Chocolate Bundt Cake

YIELD: 10 SLICES OR 6 MINI BUNDTS

1 cup plus 1 tablespoon sifted cake flour

1 small sweet potato, peeled and cubed

¼ cup low-fat buttermilk

½ cup firmly packed dark brown sugar

½ cup light corn syrup

⅛ cup vegetable oil

  1 large egg

  ½ cup unsweetened cocoa powder

  1 teaspoon baking powder

  ½ teaspoon baking soda

  ¼ teaspoon salt

  1 tablespoon confectioners' sugar

  2 ounces white chocolate, melted

1. Coat a 6-cup Bundt pan or a tray of 6 mini Bundt pans with spray oil and dust with 1 tablespoon of flour. Set aside.
2. Place the potato in a saucepan; cover with water and bring to a boil. Reduce heat and simmer, uncovered, until the potato is tender. Drain. Purée the potato in a food processor or blender. Spoon ½ cup of potato into a bowl and save or discard the remaining potato.
3. Add the buttermilk and stir until smooth. Set aside.
4. Combine the brown sugar, corn syrup, and oil in a large bowl; beat at medium speed for 5 minutes. Add the egg; beat well.
5. On a parchment paper or in a separate bowl, sift together the flour, cocoa, baking powder, baking soda, and salt; set aside. With the mixer at low speed, add the dry mixture to the creamed mixture, alternating with the potato mixture, beginning and ending with the flour mixture.
6. Pour the batter into the prepared pan. Bake at 325 degrees for 40 minutes, or until the cake springs back when lightly touched in the center. Cool for at least 15 minutes before removing from the pan. Allow the cake to cool on a cake rack.
7. Sift confectioners' sugar over the cake or drizzle melted white chocolate over individual cakes.

Nutrition Facts:

Serving size 1 slice, *or* 1/12 *a bundt cake, Calories* 184, *Fat* 3g, *Saturated Fat* 1g, *Cholesterol* 8mg, *Protein* 1g, *Carbohydrate* 42g, *Sugars* 20g, *Dietary Fiber* 0g, *Sodium* 52mg

Strawberry Shortcake

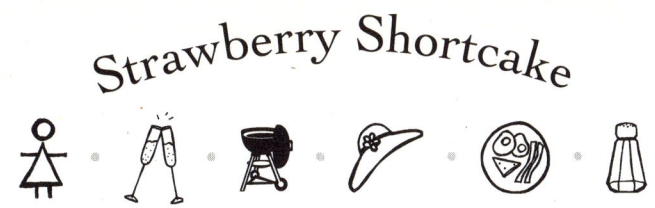

If you are short on time, you can use soft ladyfingers in place of making the shortcake. The ladyfingers are often sold by the bakery section of your supermarket.

YIELD: 6 SERVINGS

SHORTCAKE

2 cups all-purpose flour

3 tablespoons fructose

2 teaspoons baking powder

1/4 teaspoon baking soda

1/4 teaspoon salt

Zest of 1 lemon

3 tablespoons unsalted butter, chilled and sliced

3/4 cup plus 2 tablespoons low-fat buttermilk

1 egg, lightly beaten

STRAWBERRY TOPPING

2 pints fresh strawberries, sliced (4 cups)

1 tablespoon sugar

1/2 teaspoon vanilla

2 tablespoons orange juice

3/4 cup low-fat vanilla frozen yogurt

Confectioners' sugar

1. Combine the flour, fructose, baking powder and soda, salt, and zest in a bowl. Blend butter in with a large fork until the mixture resembles coarse meal. Add the buttermilk and stir until the dry ingredients are just moistened.
2. Turn the dough onto a heavily floured work area. Work the dough with your hands until you form a round ball. Do not overwork. Roll the dough to 1/2-inch thickness. Using the top of a glass or a 4-inch biscuit cutter, cut out 6 biscuits. Place the biscuits on a baking sheet lined with foil or parchment. Brush with egg and bake at 400 degrees for 15 minutes, or until light golden in color.
3. While the biscuits are baking, mix together the strawberries, sugar, vanilla, and orange juice in a large mixing bowl.

4. When the biscuits are ready, split them and place a bottom on each plate. Spoon strawberry topping onto the bottom biscuit. Top each portion with equal amounts of frozen yogurt. Cover and sprinkle tops with confectioners' sugar if desired.

Nutrition Facts:
Serving Size 1 biscuit with berries, Calories 316, Fat 8g, Saturated Fat 2g, Cholesterol 20mg, Protein 3g, Carbohydrate 20g, Sugars 7g, Dietary Fiber 1g, Sodium 108mg

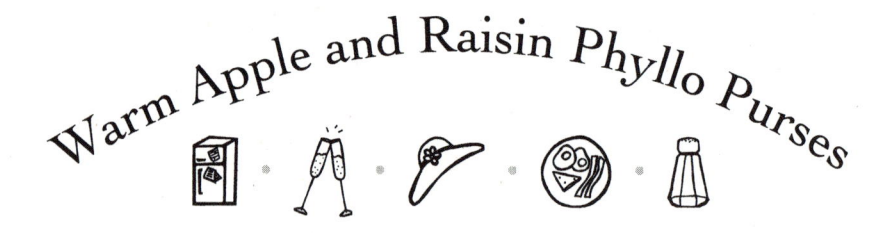

Warm Apple and Raisin Phyllo Purses

I love this recipe because of its crunchy outside crust and its comforting traditional apple pie filling. If you forgo apple pie, this makes a great substitute.

YIELD: 4 SERVINGS

½ cup apple juice concentrate

¼ cup water

2 tablespoons maple syrup

½ cup plus 1½ teaspoons cinnamon

¼ teaspoon nutmeg

⅛ teaspoon allspice

⅛ teaspoon cloves

1 teaspoon orange zest

4 Granny Smith apples, peeled and sliced ¼-inch thick

4 tablespoons golden raisins

12 sheets phyllo dough

½ cup sugar

Confectioners' sugar for topping

1. Spray a large, nonstick skillet with vegetable oil spray.
2. In a large bowl, mix together the apple juice concentrate, water, maple syrup, 1 ½ teaspoons of the cinnamon, nutmeg, allspice, cloves, and orange zest. Add the apples and raisins to this mixture and coat well. Place the mixture in the large skillet on medium heat and allow to simmer until tender and cooked about three-quarters of the way, about 5 to 10 minutes. The liquid should be evaporated. Take the apple mixture off the heat and allow to cool to room temperature.
3. Separate 12 sheets of phyllo dough from the package and keep covered with a lightly damp cloth to prevent it from drying out. Follow directions on package for working with phyllo. Using a sharp knife, cut all 12 pieces into 8-x-8-inch squares.
4. Mix together the remaining ½ cup of cinnamon and the sugar in a small bowl.
5. Each purse uses 3 sheets of phyllo. On a flat working surface place one sheet of phyllo dough, spray the sheet lightly with oil and sprinkle with the cinnamon mixture. Place the second sheet of phyllo on top of the first and repeat the process until all three sheets are bound together by the oil spray and form a square.
6. Place ¼ of the apple mixture in the center of the square. Gather the four corners of the dough together and twist. Spray the outside of the dough lightly with vegetable oil.
7. The apple purses can be frozen at this point. Otherwise, place the purses on a baking sheet lined with parchment, foil, or sprayed with oil and bake at 400 degrees until the dough is golden brown, about 10 to 15 minutes.
8. Sprinkle confectioners' sugar on top to serve. It is also nice to add a small scoop of low-fat vanilla frozen yogurt to the plate.

Nutrition Facts:
Serving Size 1 purse, *Calories* 395, *Fat* 3g, *Saturated Fat* 0g, *Cholesterol* 0mg, *Protein* 5g, *Carbohydrate* 90g, *Sugars* 54g, *Dietary Fiber* 4g, *Sodium* 280mg

Appendix I
Quick Guides for Cooking Beans and Grains

Here are charts you can make use of if you simply want to have some basic ingredients prepared and in the freezer that you can defrost and doctor up for use in recipes.

Beans

Cooking Beans

TYPE	SOAKING TIME (HOURS)	COOKING TIME & LIQUID REQUIRED	YIELD PER CUP OF BEANS
Adzuki beans	1	1 to 1½ hours in 2 cups liquid	1½
Black-eyed peas Pigeon peas	2	1 to 1½ hours in 2 cups liquid	1⅓ to 1½
Kidney, barlotti, brown, cannellini fagioli, field, flageolet, great northern, navy, pink, pinto, pearl, white	2 to 3	1 to 2 hours in 2 cups liquid	1⅓ to 1½
Black, chickpeas	3	1 to 2 hours in 2 cups liquid	1⅓ to 1½
Soybeans	Best if soaked overnight	2 hours and 25 minutes in 2 cups liquid	1½
Lentils and split Peas	None	20 to 30 minutes Lentils—1½ cups liquid Split peas—2 cups liquid	Lentils 1⅓ to 1½ Split Peas 1

Preparing the Beans for Cooking

1. Pick any stones and soil out of the beans then rinse them under cold water. Cover with water. Use 10 cups of water per pound of beans, or about three times the beans' volume in water. When you cover the beans, make sure that at least 1 inch of water reaches above them.
2. Bring to a boil for 2 minutes then remove the pot from the heat and allow the beans to soak. Remove any beans that float to the top. Note: If you prefer to do the long soaking method, you can soak the beans for twelve hours (overnight) in the refrigerator. Soak them in enough water to cover the beans by at least 1 inch.
3. When you are ready to cook the beans, drain and place them in the pot. Add enough cold broth to cover them by about 2 inches. Bring the beans slowly to a rolling boil, then turn down the heat to simmer. Skim off any foam that rises to the top of the pot.
4. Use the chart above to determine the cooking time. Add more broth if necessary. The beans should be tender but firm. If the tip of a sharp knife can easily pierce the skin, the beans are done.

Grains

When cooking grains, keep in mind that each grain has its own distinct ratio of number of cups of liquid to number of cups of grain. With a little practice, you'll learn that cooking grains is easy, and grains add great variety to meals. I encourage you to sample new grains; each one has its own distinctive texture and taste.

Cooking Grains

GRAIN	RATIO OF GRAIN/LIQUID	SIMMERING TIME IN LIQUID	YIELD
Amaranth	½ cup to ½ cup liquid	30 minutes	1½ cups
Barley Scotch barley Cracked barley	½ cup barley to 1½ cups liquid ½ cup barley to ⅓ cup liquid	45 to 55 minutes let stand 2 to 3 minutes	2 cups ⅓ cup
Buckwheat	½ cup buckwheat to 2½ cups liquid	12 minutes	2 cups
Corn Polenta Hominy	½ cup to 2 cups liquid	30 minutes	2 cups
Millet	½ cup millet to 1½ cups liquid	25 minutes	2½ cups
Oats Rolled Steel cut	½ cup grain to 1 cup liquid ½ cup grain to 2 cups liquid	5 minutes 20 minutes	1 cup 1 cup
Quinoa	½ cup grain to 1 cup liquid	15 minutes	1 cup
Rice Brown, long grain Basmati	½ cup rice to 1 cup liquid ½ cup basmati to 1½ cups liquid	For moist rice, 20 to 30 minutes 15 minutes	1½ cups 2 cups

GRAIN	RATIO OF GRAIN/LIQUID	SIMMERING TIME IN LIQUID	YIELD
Arborio	½ cup Arborio to ¾ cup liquid	15 minutes, stirring	1½ cups
Jasmine	½ cup jasmine to 1 cup liquid	15 to 20 minutes	1¾ cups
Wild	½ cup wild to 2 cups liquid	50 minutes	3 cups
Wheat Bulgur Cracked wheat	½ cup grain to 1 cup of liquid	15 to 20 minutes	1 to 1½ cups
Couscous	½ cup to ½ cup	Bring to a boil, cover and set aside 5 to 10 minutes	1 cup
Wheatberries	½ cup wheatberries to 1½ cups of liquid	1 hour and 10 minutes	1¾ cups

*Use vegetable broth instead of water to add flavor. If you are watching your sodium, look for low-sodium vegetable broth.

Appendix II
Chart of Measurements

Here are some common measurements that will be helpful in the kitchen. When measuring dry ingredients, use dry measuring cups (the short type of cup that you usually cannot see through). Spoon ingredients into cup and then level off. When measuring liquid, use a liquid measure (usually a clear large cup with a handle made of glass or plastic).

CUPS	FLUID OUNCES	TABLESPOONS	TEASPOONS	MILLILITERS
1	8	16	48	237
3/4	6	12	36	177
2/3	5 1/3	10 2/3	32	158
1/2	4	8	24	118
1/3	2 2/3	5 1/3	16	79
1/4	2	4	12	59
1/8	1	2	6	30
		1	3	15

Other Measurements to Know

Breadcrumbs (dry): 3 1/2 ounces = 1 cup
Cheese: 1 ounces = 1/4 cup grated
Dried fruit: 4 ounces = 1/2 cup
Flours: 4 ounces = 1 cup
Nuts: 2 1/2 ounces = 1/2 cup
Ground nuts: 2 ounces = 1/2 cup
Pasta and noodles
    Macaroni: 1 cup uncooked = 2 1/2 cups cooked
    Noodles: 1 cup uncooked = 1 cup cooked
    Spaghetti: 8 ounces uncooked = 4 cups cooked

Common Substitutions for Healthy Ingredients

INGREDIENT	QUANTITY	SUBSTITUTION
Low-fat buttermilk	1 cup	1 cup yogurt or 1 tablespoon lemon juice or vinegar plus enough milk to make 1 cup
Egg	1 whole (3 tablespoons)	¼ cup liquid egg substitute or 2 egg whites
Garlic	1 clove	⅛ teaspoon garlic powder
Ginger	1 teaspoon fresh	½ teaspoon ground, dried
Herbs, fresh	1 tablespoon fresh	1 teaspoon dried
Hot pepper sauce	1 teaspoon	¾ teaspoon cayenne plus 1 teaspoon vinegar
Mayonnaise, low-fat	1 cup	1 cup plain nonfat yogurt or sour cream
Mint, fresh	¼ cup chopped	1 tablespoon dried
Soy sauce	½ cup	4 tablespoons Worcestershire mixed with 1 tablespoon water
Sour cream, low fat	1 cup	1 cup nonfat or low-fat plain yogurt
Sugar	1 teaspoon	¾ teaspoon fructose or grape juice concentrate

Resources for Ingredients

Flours
Adobe Mill Company
1-800-54-Adobe
catalog of dried beans, spices

King Arthur's Flour
1-800-827-6836
www.kingarthurflour.com

Gluten Free Products
The Gluten Free Pantry, Inc.
1-203-633-3826
www.glutenfree.com
Non-gluten products for baking

Beans and Asian Products
Quality Natural Foods
1-888-392-9237
www.qualitynaturalfoods.com

Cheese
Mozzarella Company
1-800-798-2954
www.mozzarellacompany.com

Spices
Penzeys Spices
1-800-741-7787
www.penzeys.com
specialty and everyday spices

Produce
Gracewood Groves
9075 17th Place
Vero Beach, FL 32966
1-800-678-1154

Author's Note

The nutritional information for all of the recipes is taken from *Food Processor for Windows, Version 7.4*. Esha Research, Salem, OR, 1999.

While writing this book, I referenced *Cookwise* by Shirley O. Corriher (William Morrow and Company, Inc., 1997) and *Medicinal Herbs* by Penelope Ody (Dorling Kindersley, 1997).

Index

aioli, roasted red pepper, 56
almond chicken with mustard-thyme sauce, 149–50
almond oatmeal pancakes, 28–29
appetizers and party foods
   artichoke dip, 55
   avocado tomatillo salsa, 57
   cheese fondue, lite, 52
   chicken bites, Oriental, 61–62
   chicken fingers, Cajun, 63–64
   chicken saté with lite peanut sauce, 65–66
   crab cakes, 183–84
   eggplant caviar, 66–67
   hummus, 59
   mango-peach salsa, 60
   roasted red pepper aioli, 56
   shrimp skewers, Indonesian spicy, 72
   smoked salmon phyllo cups with herbed cheese spread, 58–59
   spinach pie phyllo triangles, 53–54
   tortilla cups with black bean salsa, 70–71
   vegetable spring rolls with mango-mustard sauce, classy, 68–69
apples
   baked, with yogurt and walnuts, 30–31
   butter, 29–30
   crisp, 228–29
   curry chicken with, in pita, 121–22
   in fruit combo, baked, 230–31
   and raisin phyllo purses, warm, 254–55
   in rugelach, low-fat, 247–48
apricots: about, 231
   dried, bran muffins with flaxseed and, 33–34
   in fruit combo, baked, 230–31
   ginger biscotti, 229–30
artichoke dip, 55
artichokes, steamed, in white wine broth, 218
arugula: about, 126
   salad, salmon with horseradish crust on, 193–94

Asian carrot-ginger dressing, 111
Asian marinated tuna loin, 179–80
avocados: about, 57
   and crab salad, 96–97
   tomatillo salsa, 57

balsamic vinaigrette, low-fat, 113
   garden salad with roasted vegetables and, 99–100
bananas
   bread, 32–33
   bread pudding, 231–32
   rum parfait, 233
   in waffles with fruit, healthy, 37–39
basil: about, 148
   in pesto, quick and light, 131
   and sundried tomato sauce, 137–38
   tomato shallot sauce, white sea bass in, 182
BBQ dishes
   baked tofu and vegetable wrap, 120
   beans and tofu, 134
   chicken, homestyle, 152–53

beans
  about: canned, 76; to cook, 258–59; dips, 60; protein and fiber, 85; soy, 140–41
  BBQ beans and tofu, 134
  in couscous, Moroccan spiced, 207–208
  in hummus, 59
  in jambalaya, New Orleans vegetarian, 144
  mixed, salad, 102
  mixed bean, vegetable, and cheese quesadilla, 124
  in seafood and chicken paella, lite (variation), 186–88
  three bean chili, quick and easy, 89–90
  See also specific beans
beef
  salad, Oriental, 104–106
  sirloin fajitas with peppers and onions, 169–70
  spaghetti and meatballs with baby spinach, 170–71
berries: about, 39
  crisp (variation), 228–29
  mixed, Napoleons with lemon curd, 235–36
  See also specific berries
biscotti, apricot ginger, 229–30
black bean
  salsa, tortilla cups with, 70–71
  soup, 74–75
  and spinach burritos, 135–36
blood sugar, 7–8, 12, 29, 39, 205, 235
blueberries
  cobbler, 234
  in fruit tart with cream filling, 239–40
  mixed berry Napoleons with lemon curd, 235–36
  in waffles with fruit, healthy, 37–39
blue cheese dressing, 115
bountiful burger with chipotle catsup, 167–68

breads
  banana, 32–33
  in banana bread pudding, 231–32
  bran muffins with flaxseed and dried apricots, 33–34
  in festive stuffing, low-fat, 209–10
  pancakes, almond oatmeal, 28–29
  pancakes, gingerbread, 36–37
  pancakes, traditional, 44–45
  pumpkin bread, low-fat, 41–42
  waffles with fruit, healthy, 37–39
  zucchini, 48–49
breakfast foods
  apple, baked, with yogurt and walnuts, 30–31
  apple butter, 29–30
  banana bread, 32–33
  bran muffins with flaxseed and dried apricots, 33–34
  breakfast burritos, 34–35
  chive cream cheese spread, low-fat, 39–40
  omelette, classical Spanish, 46–47
  pancakes, almond oatmeal, 28–29
  pancakes, gingerbread, 36–37
  pancakes, traditional, 44–45
  pumpkin bread, low-fat, 41–42
  quiche with spinach and tomato, low-fat, 42–44
  salmon cream cheese spread, low-fat, 40–41
  waffles with fruit, healthy, 37–39
broccoli soup, creamy, with cheddar, 77–78
broccoli with orange flavor and sesame, 217
brownie, low-fat fudge, 246–47
burger, bountiful, with chipotle catsup, 167–68

burritos, black bean and spinach, 135–36
burritos, breakfast, 34–35
butternut squash soup, roasted, 85–86

cabbage, in easy tasty fat-free or low-fat coleslaw, 98
cabbage, vegetarian stuffed, 145–46
Caesar salad, low-fat, 94
Caesar salad dressing, low-fat, 117
Cajun chicken fingers, 63–64
cakes
  cheesecake, I can't believe it's low-fat, 244–45
  chocolate bundt cake, guilt-free, 251–52
  strawberry shortcake, 253–54
calcium, 232
cantaloupe, in fruit salad with yogurt honey lime dressing, 238
carrots: about, 76
  -ginger dressing, Asian, 111
  -orange soup with ginger, 75–76
celery, apples, and walnuts, chunky chicken salad with, 95–96
cheese
  about: cheese and pasta dishes, 147; goat and sheep cheeses, 123; low-fat, 16–17
  cheddar, creamy broccoli soup with, 77–78
  cheesecake, I can't believe it's low-fat, 244–45
  cream cheese spread, low-fat salmon, 40
  in fettuccine Alfredo, lite, 206–207
  fondue, lite, 52
  goat, mixed green salad with pear and, 103–104
  herbed spread, smoked salmon phyllo cups with, 58–59

270

quesadilla, mixed bean, vegetable, and cheese, 124
ricotta and spinach stuffed shells, 142–43
in rugelach, low-fat, 247–48
in spinach lasagna, easy low-fat, 147–48
in ziti with vegetables, baked, 138–39
cheesecake, I can't believe it's low-fat, 244–45
chicken
about: fat in, 153; to roast, 133
almond, with mustard-thyme sauce, 149–50
BBQ, homestyle, 152–53
bites, Oriental, 61–62
breast, grilled marinated, 160–61
breast, sautéed, with wild mushroom sauce, 164–65
cacciatore, 154–55
curry, with apples in pita, 121–22
fingers, Cajun, 63–64
moo shu (variation), 141–42
pot pie, 155–56
roulade with crumb-nut crust, 157–58
salad, chunky, with celery, apples and walnuts, 95–96
saté with lite peanut sauce, 65–66
and seafood paella, lite, 186–88
skewers, spicy Indonesian (variation), 72
Southern-style, baked crispy, 150–52
wrap, Thai, 127–28
chickpeas
in hummus, 59
in Moroccan spiced couscous, 207–208
chili, quick and easy three bean, 89–90
chive cream cheese spread, low-fat, 39–40

chocolate: about, 247
bundt cake, guilt-free, 251–52
in fudge brownie, low-fat, 246–47
oatmeal chocolate chip cookies, 249–50
pudding, homemade fat-free, 242
cobbler, blueberry, 234
coleslaw, easy tasty fat-free or low-fat, 98
condiments. See sauces
cookies
apricot ginger biscotti, 229–30
fudge brownie, low-fat, 246–47
oatmeal chocolate chip, 249–50
rugelach, low-fat, 247–48
corn chowder, decadent, 78–79
couscous: to cook, 261
Moroccan spiced, 207–208
crab
and avocado salad, 96–97
cakes, 183–84
topping for decadent corn chowder (optional), 79
cranberries
-orange sauce, spiced pork medallions with, 177–79
in rugelach, low-fat, 247–48
in wheatberry salad with raspberry vinaigrette, 213–14
curry
chicken with apples in pita, 121–22
grilled scallops, spicy, with mango mint salsa, 195–96
-orange tofu with vegetables, baked, 139–40

dairy, about: buttermilk, 112; calcium, 232; goat and sheep cheeses, 123; low-fat cheeses, 16–17; yogurt, 122, 239
decadent corn chowder, 78–79
desserts
apple and raisin phyllo purses, warm, 254–55

apple crisp, 228–29
apricot ginger biscotti, 229–30
banana bread pudding, 231–32
banana rum parfait, 233
blueberry cobbler, 234
cheesecake, I can't believe it's low-fat, 244–45
chocolate bundt cake, guilt-free, 251–52
chocolate pudding, homemade fat-free, 242
fruit combo, baked, 230–31
fruit salad with yogurt honey lime dressing, 238
fruit tart with cream filling, 239–40
fudge brownie, low-fat, 246–47
lemon tart, 243–44
mixed berry Napoleons with lemon curd, 235–36
oatmeal chocolate chip cookies, 249–50
oranges, glazed Venetian, 241
raspberry soufflés, 250–51
rugelach, low-fat, 247–48
strawberry shortcake, 253–54
dips
about: premade, 67; as snack, 60; vegetable-based, 56
artichoke, 55
eggplant caviar, 66–67
hummus, 59
roasted red pepper aioli, 56
See also salsa; spreads
dressings. See salad dressings
duck: about, 160
breast with port wine sauce, 159–60

eggplant caviar, 66–67
eggs: about, 35
in breakfast burritos, 34–35
in omelette, classic Spanish, 46–47
in quiche with spinach and tomato, low-fat, 42–44

271

fajitas, sirloin, with peppers and onions, 169–70
fats, about: avocados, 57; eggs, 35; list of, 11–12; nuts, 96; poultry, 153, 160
festive stuffing, low-fat, 209–10
fettuccine Alfredo, lite, 206–207
fish, about: mercury, 180–81; PCBs, 193; to roast, 133
See also specific types of fish
flaxseed and dried apricots, bran muffins with, 33–34
fondue, lite cheese, 52
fructose, 235
fruits
　about: adding to pancakes, 45; apricots, 231; disease prevention, 31; mangos, 60; nutrients, 13–14; pesticides, 15
　combo, baked, 230–31
　dried, pork loin stuffed with, 176–77
　in lamb stew, Moroccan, 173–74
　salad with yogurt honey lime dressing, 238
　tart with cream filling, 239–40
　waffles with, healthy, 37–39
　See also specific fruits

gazpacho soup, 80–81
gingerbread pancakes, 36–37
goat cheese, mixed green salad with pear and, 103–104
grains and starches, about: to cook, 259–61; nut and grain combinations, 29; nutrients, 12–13; refined flour, 152
　See also specific grains or starches
gravy, sherry cider, roast turkey with, 162–64
Greek salad, low-fat, 100–101
green beans
　and toasted pine nuts, new potato salad with, 210–11

greens
　about: arugula, 126; dark leafy vegetables, 221
　in garden salad with roasted vegetables and balsamic dressing, 99–100
　with garlic, sautéed, 220
　mixed green salad with pear and goat cheese, 103–104
　See also spinach

halibut, potato-crusted, with white wine sauce, 190–91
herbs and spices
　about: basil, 148; cinnamon, 248; flavoring with, 21–22, 130–33; ginger, 37; herbs de Provence, 176; parsley, 103; thyme, 197
　for bouquet garni, 73–74
　in gingerbread pancakes, 36–37
　herbed cheese spread, smoked salmon phyllo cups with, 58–59
　herb-roasted salmon over caramelized leeks, 185–86
　herbs and garlic, rack of lamb with, 175
　herb vinaigrette, fresh, 116
　Indian spices, spinach with, 219
　Moroccan spiced couscous, 207–208
　spice rub: for Cajun chicken fingers, 63; for spiced pork medallions, 178
　See also specific herbs
honeydew, in fruit salad with yogurt honey lime dressing, 238
honey mustard dipping sauce, 151
honey-mustard dressing, 114–15
hors d'oeuvres. *See* appetizers and party foods
hummus, 59; roasted vegetable sandwich with, 125–26

I can't believe it's low-fat cheesecake, 244–45
Indian spices, spinach with, 219
Indonesian shrimp skewers, 72
Italian roasted portabello sandwich, 122–23

jambalaya, New Orleans vegetarian, 144

lamb, rack of, with herbs and garlic, 175
lamb stew, Moroccan, 173–74
lasagna, easy low-fat spinach, 147–48
leeks, caramelized, herb-roasted salmon over, 185–86
lemon
　curd, mixed berry Napoleons with, 235–36
　-tarragon buttermilk dressing, 112; roasted salmon salad with, 106–107
　tart, 243–44
lentil salad, warm, 109
lentil soup, 84–85
lime dressing, creamy, salmon with, 192
lime yogurt honey dressing, fruit salad with, 238

mangos: about, 60
　mint salsa, spicy curry grilled scallops with, 195–96
　-mustard sauce, classy vegetable spring rolls with, 68–69
　-peach salsa, 60
　salsa, shrimp with, 108
marinades: about, 130
　for Asian marinated tuna loin, 179–80
　for grilled marinated chicken breast, 160–61
　for grilled vegetables, 200
　orange-curry, 139–40
　for sirloin fajitas with peppers and onions, 169–70

for spiced pork medallions, 177–79
Thai, 127–28
measurements, 263–64
meatballs and spaghetti with baby spinach, 170–71
meat loaf, traditional turkey, 166–67
meats, lean, 15–16, 168
See also specific types of meat
Mediterranean roasted red pepper soup, 87–88
mint mango salsa, spicy curry grilled scallops with, 195–96
monkfish, in lite seafood and chicken paella, 186–88
moo shu, soy, 141–42
Moroccan lamb stew, 173–74
Moroccan spiced couscous, 207–208
muffins
   banana bread (variation), 32–33
   bran muffins with flaxseed and dried apricots, 33–34
   low-fat pumpkin bread (variation), 41–42
   zucchini bread, 48–49
mushrooms: about, 82
   portabello sandwich, Italian roasted, 122–23
   -shallot soup, rich and elegant, 81–82
   wild mushroom sauce, sautéed chicken breast with, 164–65
mustard
   honey dipping sauce, 151
   -honey salad dressing, 114–15
   -mango sauce, vegetable spring rolls with, classy, 68–69
   -thyme sauce, almond chicken with, 149–50

Napoleons, mixed berry, with lemon curd, 235–36
New Orleans vegetarian jambalaya, 144

noodles, sesame, 211–12
nuts, about: daily servings, 66; fats in, 96; nut and grain combinations, 29; to toast, 104
See also specific nuts

oatmeal
   almond pancakes, 28–29
   chocolate chip cookies, 249–50
   in traditional pancakes, 44–45
omelette, classic Spanish, 46–47
oranges and orange juice
   broccoli with orange flavor and sesame, 217
   -carrot soup with ginger, 75–76
   -cranberry sauce, spiced pork medallions with, 177–79
   -curry tofu with vegetables, baked, 139–40
   in fruit salad with yogurt honey lime dressing, 238
   glazed Venetian, 241
organic foods, about: flavor, 13; pesticides, 15; USDA labeling, 17–18
Oriental beef salad, 104–106
Oriental chicken bites, 61–62

paella, lite seafood and chicken, 186–88
pancakes
   almond oatmeal, 28–29
   gingerbread, 36–37
   traditional, 44–45
parfait, banana rum, 233
party foods. *See* appetizers and party foods
pasta
   about: cheese and pasta dishes, 147; couscous, 208, 261
   couscous, Moroccan spiced, 207–208
   fettuccine Alfredo, lite, 206–207
   lasagna, easy low-fat spinach, 147–48
   noodles, sesame, 211–12

   shells, spinach and ricotta stuffed, 143
   spaghetti and meatballs with baby spinach, 170–71
   ziti with vegetables, baked, 138–39
peaches
   crisp (variation), 228–29
   in fruit tart with cream filling, 239–40
   -mango salsa, 60
   in shrimp with mango salsa, 108
peanut butter: about, 13
   peanut sauce, lite, chicken saté with, 65–66
   in sesame noodles, 211–12
pears
   crisp (variation), 228–29
   in fruit combo, baked, 230–31
   and goat cheese, mixed green salad with, 103–104
pecan-cornmeal crust, trout with, 196–97
peppers. *See* red peppers
pesto: about, 130–31
   quick and light, 131
   quinoa with, 216
phyllo
   for chicken pot pie, 156–57
   cups, smoked salmon, with herbed cheese spread, 58–59
   for mixed berry Napoleons with lemon curd, 235–36
   purses, warm apple and raisin, 254–55
   for vegetable strudel with red pepper sauce, 221–23
pineapple
   in baked orange-curry tofu with vegetables, 139–40
   in fruit salad with yogurt honey lime dressing, 238
   in shrimp with mango salsa (variation), 108
pine nuts, toasted, new potato salad with green beans and, 210–11

pistachios
   in chicken roulade with crumb-nut crust, 157–58
   in glazed Venetian oranges (option), 241
   in mixed berry Napoleons with lemon curd, 235–36
plums, in baked fruit combo, 230–31
pork loin stuffed with dried fruit, 176–77
pork medallions, spiced, with cranberry-orange sauce, 177–79
portabello sandwich, Italian roasted, 122–23
port wine sauce, duck breast with, 159–60
potatoes: about, 205
   -crusted halibut with white wine sauce, 190–91
   fries, baked, 204
   roasted new, easy, 203
   salad, new, with green beans and toasted pine nuts, 210–11
   Yukon gold mashed, 205–06
pot pie, chicken, 155–56
poultry. *See specific types of poultry*
Provençal, vegetables gratin, 223–24
pudding, banana bread, 231–32
pudding, homemade fat-free chocolate, 242
pumpkin bread, low-fat, 41–42
puttenesca sauce, tilapia in, 184–85

quesadilla, mixed bean, vegetable, and cheese, 124
quiche with spinach and tomato, low-fat, 42–44
quinoa with pesto, 216

raspberries
   coulis, 237
   in mixed berry Napoleons with lemon curd, 235–36

   soufflés, 250–51
   vinaigrette, 114
   vinaigrette, wheatberry salad with, 213–14
   in waffles with fruit, healthy, 213–14
red peppers: about, 88
   aioli, roasted, 56
   and onions, sirloin fajitas with, 169–70
   sauce, vegetable strudel with, 221–23
   soup, Mediterranean roasted, 87–88
   tapenade, sundried tomato–roasted red pepper, 132
rhubarb crisp (variation), 228–29
rice: to cook, 260–61
   pilaf, wild and brown, 214–15
   in vegetarian jambalaya, New Orleans, 144
rich and elegant mushroom-shallot soup, 81–82
ricotta and spinach stuffed shells, 143
roast, how to, 133
rugelach, low-fat, 247–48

salad dressings
   balsamic vinaigrette, low-fat, 113
   blue cheese, 115
   Caesar salad, low-fat, 117
   carrot-ginger, Asian, 111
   herb vinaigrette, fresh, 116
   honey-mustard, 114–15
   lemon-tarragon buttermilk, 112
   lime, creamy, 192
   raspberry vinaigrette, 114, 213–14
   yogurt honey lime, 238
salads
   arugula, salmon with horseradish crust on, 193–94
   bean, mixed, 102

   beef, Oriental, 104–106
   Caesar, low-fat, 94
   chicken, chunky, with celery, apples and walnuts, 95–96
   coleslaw, easy tasty fat-free or low-fat, 98
   crab and avocado, 96–97
   fruit, with yogurt honey lime dressing, 238
   garden, with roasted vegetables and balsamic dressing, 99–100
   Greek, low-fat, 100–101
   green, mixed, with pear and goat cheese, 103–104
   lentil, warm, 109
   salmon, roasted, with lemon-tarragon buttermilk dressing, 106–107
   shrimp with mango salsa, 108
   wheatberry, with raspberry vinaigrette, 213–14
salmon
   cream cheese spread, low-fat, 40–41
   with creamy lime dressing, 192
   herb-roasted, over caramelized leeks, 185–86
   with horseradish crust on arugula salad, 193–94
   salad, roasted, with lemon-tarragon buttermilk dressing, 106–107
   smoked salmon phyllo cups with herbed cheese spread, 58–59
salsa
   avocado tomatillo, 57
   black bean, 70
   mango, 108
   mango mint, 195–96
   mango-peach, 60
sandwiches
   BBQ baked tofu and vegetable wrap, 120
   chicken wrap, Thai, 127–28

curry chicken with apples in pita, 121–22
mixed bean, vegetable, and cheese quesadilla, 124
portabello, Italian roasted, 122–23
vegetable, roasted, with hummus, 125–26
sauces: about, 143
   BBQ, 152–53
   chipotle catsup, 167–68
   cilantro sour cream, 63–64
   cranberry-orange, 178
   curry yogurt, 121
   honey mustard dipping sauce, 151
   mango-mustard, 68–69
   mustard-thyme, 149–50
   for Oriental chicken bites, 61–62
   peanut, 65–66
   pesto, quick and light, 131
   port wine, 159
   puttenesca, 184–85
   raspberry coulis, 237
   red pepper, 221–23
   sesame, 212
   sherry cider gravy, 162
   sundried tomato and basil, 137–38
   tomato basil shallot, 182
   wasabi, 179–80
   white wine, 190–91
   wild mushroom, 165
   See also salsa
scallops
   in seafood and chicken paella, lite, 186–88
   skewers, spicy Indonesian (variation), 72
   spicy curry grilled, with mango mint salsa, 195–96
seafood and chicken paella, lite, 186–88
sesame and orange flavor, broccoli with, 217
sesame noodles, 211–12
shellfish. *See specific types of shellfish*

sherry cider gravy, roast turkey with, 162–64
shortcake, strawberry, 253–54
shrimp
   Creole, lite, 188–89
   with mango salsa, 108
   moo shu (variation), 141–42
   in seafood and chicken paella, lite, 186–88
   skewers, spicy Indonesian, 72
sirloin fajitas with peppers and onions, 169–70
soufflés, raspberry, 250–51
soups
   black bean, 74–75
   broccoli with cheddar, creamy, 77–78
   butternut squash, roasted, 85–86
   carrot-orange, with ginger, 75–76
   corn chowder, decadent, 78–79
   gazpacho, 80–81
   lentil, 84–85
   mushroom-shallot, rich and elegant, 81–82
   roasted red pepper, Mediterranean, 87–88
   sweet pea, 88–89
   three bean chili, quick and easy, 89–90
   vegetable, hearty, 83–84
   white bean, 90–91
Southern-style chicken, baked crispy, 150–52
soy: benefits of, 140–41
   moo shu, 141–42
   in vegetarian stuffed cabbage, 145
   See also tofu
spaghetti and meatballs with baby spinach, 170–71
spanikopita, 53–54
spiced pork medallions with cranberry-orange sauce, 177–79
spices. *See* herbs and spices

spinach
   baby, meatballs and spaghetti with, 170–71
   and black bean burritos, 135–36
   with Indian spices, 219
   lasagna, easy low-fat, 147–48
   pie phyllo triangles, 53–54
   and ricotta stuffed shells, 143
   and tomato, low-fat quiche with, 42–44
spreads
   about: for flavor enhancement, 132; jams and preserves, 45
   apple butter, 29–30
   chive cream cheese, low-fat, 39–40
   herbed cheese, 58–59
   roasted red pepper aioli, 56
   salmon cream cheese, low-fat, 40–41
   See also dips
spring rolls with mango-mustard sauce, classy vegetable, 68–69
squash soup, roasted butternut, 85–86
starches. *See* grains and starches, about; *specific grains or starches*
stew, Moroccan lamb, 173–74
strawberries
   in fruit salad with yogurt honey lime dressing, 238
   in fruit tart with cream filling, 239–40
   in mixed berry Napoleons with lemon curd, 235–36
   shortcake, 253–54
   in waffles with fruit, healthy, 37–39
strudel, vegetable, with red pepper sauce, 221–23
stuffing, festive low-fat, 209–10
substitutions, common, 265
sundried tomato and basil sauce, 137–38

sundried tomato–roasted red pepper tapenade, 132
sunflower seeds, about, 49
sweet pea soup, 88–89
sweet potatoes, for baked potato fries, 204

tapenade: for flavor enhancement, 130–31
    sundried tomato–roasted red pepper, 132
tart, lemon, 243
Thai chicken wrap, 127–28
three bean chili, quick and easy, 89–90
tilapia in puttenesca sauce, 184–85
tofu
    BBQ beans and, 134
    for honey-mustard dressing, 114–15
    in jambalaya, New Orleans vegetarian, 144
    in paella, lite (variation), 186–88
    skewers, spicy Indonesian (variation), 72
    with vegetables, baked orange-curry, 139–40
    in vegetable spring rolls with mango-mustard sauce, classy, 68–69
    and vegetable wrap, BBQ baked, 120
tomatillo avocado salsa, 57
tomato
    basil shallot sauce, white sea bass in, 182
    and spinach, low-fat quiche with, 42–44
    sundried, and basil sauce, 137–38
    sundried–roasted red pepper tapenade, 132
toppings. *See* sauces; spreads
tortilla cups with black bean salsa, 70–71

trout with pecan-cornmeal crust, 196–97
tuna loin, Asian marinated, 179–80
turkey: to roast, 133
    in bountiful burger with chipotle catsup, 167–68
    meat loaf, traditional, 166–67
    roast, with sherry cider gravy, 162–64
    roulade with crumb-nut crust (variation), 157–58

veal Marsala, 172–73
vegetables
    about: asparagus, 107; to cook, 199–202; cruciferous, 99, 126; in dips, 56; horseradish root, 194; nutrients, 13–15; onions, 110; orange-colored, 42, 76; as part of dinner, 149; pesticides, 15; potatoes and sweet potatoes, 205
    in gazpacho soup, 80–81
    gratin Provençal, 223–24
    mixed bean, vegetable, and cheese quesadilla, 124
    orange-curry tofu with, baked, 139–40
    roasted, 224–25
    roasted vegetables, garden salad with, and balsamic dressing, 99–100
    roasted vegetable sandwich with hummus, 125–26
    soup, hearty, 83–84
    spring rolls with mango-mustard sauce, classy, 68–69
    strudel with red pepper sauce, 221–23
    wrap, BBQ baked tofu and, 120
    ziti with, baked, 138–39
    See also salads; *specific vegetables*

Venetian oranges, glazed, 241
vinaigrettes. *See* salad dressings

walnuts
    baked apple with yogurt and, 30–31
    chunky chicken salad with celery, apples and, 95–96
    in low-fat festive stuffing (option), 209–10
wasabi sauce, for Asian marinated tuna loin, 179–80
weight loss, 6–10
wheatberries: to cook, 261
    salad with raspberry vinaigrette, 213–14
white bean soup, 90–91
white sea bass in tomato basil shallot sauce, 182
white wine broth, steamed artichokes in, 218
white wine sauce, potato-crusted halibut with, 190–91
wild and brown rice pilaf, 214–15
wild mushroom sauce, sautéed chicken breast with, 164–65
wrap sandwiches: about, 126–27
    BBQ baked tofu and vegetable, 120
    Thai chicken, 127–28

yogurt: about, 122, 239
    honey lime dressing, fruit salad with, 238
    and walnuts, baked apple with, 30–31
Yukon gold mashed potatoes, 205–206

ziti with vegetables, baked, 138–39
zucchini bread, 48–49